2012-2013

HESI Live Review Workbook for the NCLEX-RN® Exam

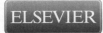

ELSEVIER

3251 Riverport Lane
St. Louis, MO 63043

2012-2013 HESI Live
Review Workbook for the NCLEX-RN® Exam

ISBN: 978-1-4557-0645-7

NOTICE

Knowledge and best practice in this field are constantly changing. As new research and experience broaden our understanding, changes in research methods, professional practices, or medical treatment may become necessary.

Practitioners and researchers must always rely on their own experience and knowledge in evaluating and using any information, methods, compounds, or experiments described herein. In using such information or methods they should be mindful of their own safety and the safety of others, including parties for whom they have a professional responsibility.

With respect to any drug or pharmaceutical products identified, readers are advised to check the most current information provided (i) on procedures featured or (ii) by the manufacturer of each product to be administered, to verify the recommended dose or formula, the method and duration of administration, and contraindications. It is the responsibility of practitioners, relying on their own experience and knowledge of their patients, to make diagnoses, to determine dosages and the best treatment for each individual patient, and to take all appropriate safety precautions.

To the fullest extent of the law, neither the Publisher nor the authors, contributors, or editors, assume any liability for any injury and/or damage to persons or property as a matter of products liability, negligence or otherwise, or from any use or operation of any methods, products, instructions, or ideas contained in the material herein.

The Publisher

NCLEX®, NCLEX-RN®, and NCLEX-PN® are registered trademarks of the National Council of State Boards of Nursing, Inc.

International Standard Book Number: 978-1-4557-0645-7

Executive Editor: Kristin Geen
Developmental Editor: Lauren Harms
Publishing Services Manager: Jeffrey Patterson
Project Manager: Siva Raman Krishnamoorthy
Design Direction: Jessica Williams

Printed in the United States of America

Last digit is the print number: 9   8   7   6   5   4   3

Working together to grow
libraries in developing countries

www.elsevier.com | www.bookaid.org | www.sabre.org

ELSEVIER   BOOK AID International   Sabre Foundation

Contributing Authors

Susan Morrison, PhD, RN
President Emerita
Elsevier Review and Testing
Nursing and Health Professions
Houston, Texas

Ainslie Nibert, PhD, RN
Vice President
Elsevier Review and Testing
Nursing and Health Professions
Houston, Texas

Mickie Hinds, PhD, RN
Director, Review and Curriculum
Elsevier Review and Testing
Nursing and Health Professions
Houston, Texas

Judy R. Hyland, MS, RN
Manager, Review and Curriculum
Elsevier Review and Testing
Nursing and Health Professions
Houston, Texas

Judy Siefert, MSN, RN
Director, Testing
Elsevier Review and Testing
Nursing and Health Professions
Houston, Texas

Denise Voyles, BSN, RN
Testing Manager
Elsevier Review and Testing
Nursing and Health Professions
Houston, Texas

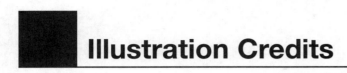# Illustration Credits

Chapter 7: Movement, Coordination, and Sensory Input
From Lewis, S., Heitkemper, M., Dirksen, S., O'Brien, P., & Bucher, L. (2007). *Medical-surgical nursing: Assessment and management of clinical problems* (7th ed.). St Louis: Mosby.

Chapter 9: Maternal-Newborn Nursing
From Lowdermilk, D., & Perry, S. (2007). *Maternity and women's health care* (9th ed.). St Louis: Mosby.

Contents

1 Test-Taking Strategies and Study Guide

WELCOME TO THE HESI LIVE REVIEW COURSE

This series of slides and the workbook provide test-taking strategies and a content review of nursing curriculum to help prepare nursing students for the NCLEX-RN examination. If students want a more in-depth review of certain material please refer to:

- *HESI Comprehensive Review for the NCLEX-RN Examination*
- *Mosby's Comprehensive Review of Nursing for NCLEX-RN Examination*
- *Saunders Comprehensive Review for the NCLEX-RN Examination*

Knowledge Is Power!

- Enhance test-taking skills
- Review basic curriculum content
- Organize knowledge
- Identify content weakness
- Know what to expect
- Manage anxiety
- Establish study plan

NLCEX-RN EXAMINATION

- Safe and Effective Practice
- "Essential" Nursing Knowledge
- **Think: safety, *safety,* SAFETY!**

Nursing Process

- Planning and implementing nursing care based on assessment, diagnosis, and determining priorities
- Evaluating the effectiveness of nursing care

Client Needs

- Safe and effective care environment
- Management of care
  — Safety and infection control
- Health promotion and maintenance
- Psychosocial integrity
- Physiological integrity
  — Basic care and comfort
  — Pharmacological and parenteral therapies
  — Reduction of risk potential
  — Physiological adaptation

- The test plan is revised every 3 years after conducting a practice analysis with entry-level nurses.
- Information about the test plan, including descriptions of content categories and related content for each category, can be found at **www.ncsbn.org**.
- This site also contains information for students, frequently asked questions, and examples of alternate formats.

TEST-TAKING STRATEGIES

- ABCs
- Maslow's Hierarchy of Needs
- Start with least invasive intervention
- Assess before taking action, when appropriate
- Have all the necessary information/take all possible relevant actions before calling the physician/health-care provider
- Which client to assess first (most at risk, most physiologically unstable)

Strategies for Success: Four Essential Steps

1. Determine if the style of the question is

+ positive +

or

− negative −

2. Find the key words in the question
3. Rephrase the question in your own words and answer the question
4. Rule out options

Determine if the Question Is Written in a Positive or Negative Style

- A *positive style* may ask what the nurse should do, or the best or first action to implement.
- A *negative style* may ask what the nurse should avoid, which prescription the nurse should question, or which behavior indicates the need for reteaching the client.

Find the Key Words in the Question

- Ask yourself which words or phrases provide the critical information?
- This information may be the age of the client, the setting, the timing, a set of symptoms or behaviors, or any number of other factors.
- For example, the nursing actions for a 10-year-old, 1-day postoperative client are different from those for a 70-year-old, 1-hour postoperative client.

Rephrase the Question in Your Own Words

- This will help you eliminate nonessential information in the question and help you determine the correct answer.
- Ask yourself, "What is this instructor *really* asking?"
- Before looking at the choices, rephrase the question in your own words.
- Answer the question.

2

Rule out options
- Based on your knowledge, you can probably identify one or two options that are clearly incorrect.
- Mentally mark through those options on the computer monitor.
- Now, differentiate between the remaining options, considering your knowledge of the subject and related nursing principles, such as roles of the nurse, nursing process, ABCs, and Maslow's Hierarchy of Needs.

A client who has COPD is resting in a semi-Fowler's position with oxygen at 2 L/min per nasal cannula. The client develops dyspnea. What action should the nurse implement first?
A. Call the healthcare provider
B. Obtain a bedside pulse oximeter
C. Raise the head of the bed farther
D. Assess the client's vital signs

The Question May Contain *"Red Flag Words."*
Practice rewording the questions below:
1. "Which response indicates to the nurse a need to *reteach* the client about …"
2. "Which prescription (order) should the nurse *question?*"

Common interventions include:
- Small, frequent feedings
- Recommended fluid intake: "3 L/day"
- Alternate rest with activity
- Conserve energy with any activity

TEACHING POINTS
- Risk factors: known modifiable vs. nonmodifiable
- Prevention and wellness promotion
- New medications/self-care instructions
- Client empowerment
- *Anticipatory* guidance
- Incorporating within the client's **lifestyle, culture, spiritual beliefs,** etc.

A Few Words About "Words"
- Healthcare provider: the person prescribing care (e.g., physician, nurse practitioner)
  — Physician = "doctor"
  — Prescriptions = "orders"
- Unlicensed assistive personnel
  — Patient care technician
  — Nursing assistant
  — Nurse's aide

Keep Memorizing to a Minimum
- Growth and developmental milestones
- Death and dying stages
- Crisis intervention

[handwritten: DABDA]

[handwritten: do not teach new coping styles when pt in crisis]

HESI Test Question Approach			
Positive?		YES	NO
Key Words			
Rephrase			
Rule Out Choices			
A	B	C	D

[handwritten: "When the pt is in distress don't assess"]

- Immunizations
- Drug classifications
- Principles of teaching/learning
- Stages of pregnancy and fetal growth
- Nurse Practice Act: Standards of Practice & Delegation

Know Normal Ranges for Commonly Used Lab Tests (Appendix A), What Variations Mean, and the Best Nursing Actions
- H & H
- WBC, RBC, platelets   *9–10.5*
- Electrolytes: K^+, Na^+, Ca^{2+}, Mg^{2+}, Cl^-, PO_4^-
- BUN and creatinine
- *Relationship* of Ca^{2+} and PO_4^-
- ABGs
- PT, INR, PTT (don't get them confused)

Warfarin   Heparin

A client who has hyperparathyroidism is scheduled to receive a prescribed dose of oral phosphate. The nurse notes that the client's serum calcium level is 12.5 mg/dL. What action should the nurse implement?
A. Hold the phosphate and notify the healthcare provider
B. Review the client's serum parathyroid hormone level
C. Give a PRN dose of IV calcium per protocol
D. Administer the dose of oral phosphate

ALTERNATE FORMAT QUESTIONS

The NCLEX is primarily single response multiple choice questions. However, it will be helpful to have a basic familiarity of the alternate test format questions you may encounter. The current types include:
- Fill-in-the-blank
- Exhibit
- Audio
- Multiple response
- Hot spot
- Drag and drop

NUTRITION

Be able to identify foods relative to their sodium content (high or low), potassium levels (high or low), and increased levels of phosphate, iron, or vitamin K
- Chemotherapy, GI/GU disturbances
- Proteins, CHOs, fats
- Pregnancy and fetal growth needs
- Remember concepts:
    — Introducing one food at a time (infants, allergies)
    — Progression "AS TOLERATED"
- What nursing assessment guides decisions regarding progression?

HESI Test Question Approach		
Positive?	YES	NO
Key Words		
Rephrase		
Rule Out Choices		
A	B	C	D

$$\frac{250\,ml}{60\,min} \times \frac{15\,drops}{ml} = 63$$

MEDICATION ADMINISTRATION AND PHARMACOLOGY

Pharmacological treatment and related nursing implications will be reviewed in each chapter to coincide with the disease processes and conditions of the client.

More critical thinking questions are being designed around SKILLS!

Think: safety, *safety*, SAFETY!

Reflect on … the *Whole Picture*

Safe medication administration is more than just knowing the action of the medications:

- "6 Rights"—five *plus* technique of skill execution
- Drug interactions
- Vulnerable organs: ✓labs; what to assess
- Allergies and presence of suprainfections
- Concept of peak and trough
- How you would know:
    — It's working
    — There's a problem
- Teaching: *safety, empowerment, compliance*

Special Considerations

- Teratogens – harmful to fetus
- Vesicants ~~irritant~~ to tissue/vessels –
- Implications of edema, impaired tissue perfusion of injection site
- Hepatorenal status to drug dose/frequency
- Concepts of weaning

Cautionary Tales

Do Not Respond Based on …

- *Your* past client care experiences or agency
- A familiar phrase or term
- "Of course, *I* would have already …"
- What *you* think is *realistic*
- *Your* children, pregnancies, parents, elders, personal response to a drug, etc.

Do respond based on …

- ABCs
- Scientific, behavioral, sociologic principles
- Principles of teaching/learning
- Maslow's Hierarchy
- Nursing process
- What's in the stem: no more, no less
- NCLEX-RN ideal hospital
- Basic A&P
- Critical thinking

STUDY GUIDE: TAKE CARE OF YOURSELF

From Now Until the Test:

- *Do* set up a study schedule and stick to it
- *Do* avoid negative people
- *Do* respect your body and your mind
- *Do* think positively—say to yourself, "*I can be successful!*"

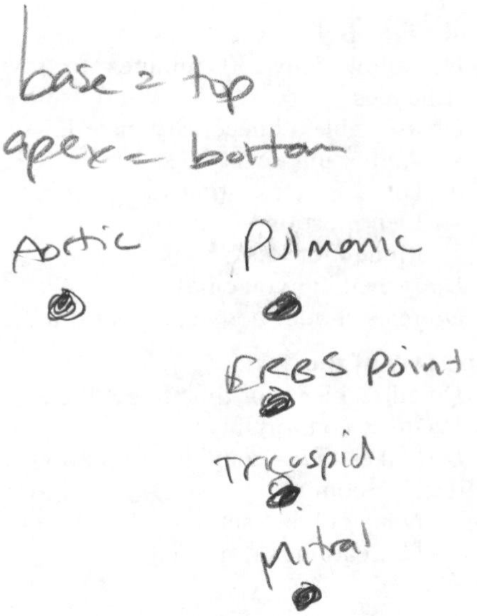

[Handwritten margin notes:]

base = top
apex = bottom

Aortic   Pulmonic

Erbs point

Tricuspid

Mitral

Pregnancy – heparin

teaching → empower client immediate feedback?

The Night Before the Test:

- *Do* allow only 30 minutes to review test-taking strategies
- *Do* assemble all necessary materials
  — Admission ticket
  — Directions to testing center
  — Identification
  — Money for lunch
- *Do* something you enjoy
- *Do* respect your body and your mind

The Day of the Test:

- *Do* allow plenty of time to get there
- *Do* dress comfortably
- *Do* take *only* your identification forms into the testing room
  — *Do* avoid distractions
  — Use earplugs if needed

2 Legal Issues, Acute Conditions, Disaster Management, and Bioterrorism

LEGAL ISSUES

Legal Systems
- Civil law is concerned with the protection of the client's private rights
- Criminal law deals with the rights of individuals and society as defined by legislative laws

Nursing malpractice: The failure to use that degree of care that a reasonable nurse would use under the same or similar circumstances.
- Malpractice is founded when:
- The nurse owed a duty to the client
- The nurse did not carry out that duty or breached that duty
- The client was injured
- The nurse's failure to carry out that duty caused the client's injury

Standards of Care
- Nurses are required to follow standards of care, which originate in Nurse Practice Acts, the guidelines of professional organizations.
- Nurses are required to follow written policies and procedures of employing institutions.
- Nurses are responsible for performing procedures correctly and exercising professional judgment when you carry out healthcare provider prescriptions.

The unlicensed assistive personnel (UAP) reports to a staff nurse that a client, who had surgery 4 hours ago, has a decrease in blood pressure (BP) from 150/80 to 110/70 in the last hour. The nurse advises the UAP to check the client's dressing for excess drainage and report the findings to the nurse. Which factor is most important to consider when assessing the legal ramifications of this situation?
A. The parameters of the state's nurse practice act
B. The need to complete an adverse occurrence report
C. Hospital protocols regarding the frequency of vital sign assessment every hour postoperatively
D. The physician's prescription regarding changing the postoperative dressing

Practice Issues
- Nurses must follow the healthcare provider's prescriptions unless the nurse believes that it is in error, violates hospital policy, or is harmful to the patient.
- The nurse will make a formal report explaining the refusal.

Malpractice = harm is caused (handwritten)

HESI Test Question Approach			
Positive?		YES	NO
Key Words			
Rephrase			
Rule Out Choices			
A	B	C	D

- The nurse should file an incident (occurrence) report in any situation that will potentially cause harm to a patient.

Advance Directives (AD)
- Assess client's knowledge of AD
- Integrate AD into client plan of care
- Provide client with information about AD

Restraints

A family member of a female client who is in a Posey vest restraint asks why the restraint was applied. How should the nurse respond?

A. This restraint was prescribed by the healthcare provider.

B. There is not enough staff to keep her safe all the time.

C. The other patients are upset when she wanders at night.

D. Her actions place her at high risk for harming herself.

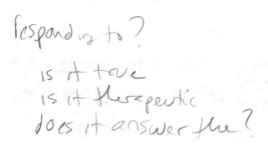
responding to?
is it true
is it therapeutic
does it answer the?

HESI Test Question Approach			
Positive?		YES	NO
Key Words			
Rephrase			
Rule Out Choices			
A	B	C	D

Psychiatric Nursing
- Admissions
  — Involuntary
  — Emergency
- Client rights
- Competency

What nursing action has the highest priority when admitting a client to a psychiatric unit on an involuntary basis?

A. Reassure the client that this admission is only for a limited amount of time.

B. Offer the client and family the opportunity to share their feelings about the admission.

C. Determine the behaviors that resulted in the need for admission.

D. Advise the client about the legal rights of all hospitalized clients.

HESI Test Question Approach			
Positive?		YES	NO
Key Words			
Rephrase			
Rule Out Choices			
A	B	C	D

Confidential Healthcare
- All clients are protected under the Health Insurance Portability and Accountability Act of 1996 (HIPAA)
  — HIPAA sets standards regarding the verbal written and electronic exchange of private health information.
  — HIPAA creates client rights to consent to use and disclose health information, to inspect and copy one's medical record, and to amend mistaken or incomplete information.

8

— The standards require all hospitals and health agencies to have specific policies and procedures in place to ensure compliance with the standards.

Informed Consent

Informed consent must meet the following criteria:

- The client giving consent is competent and of legal age
- The consent is given voluntarily
- The client giving consent understands the procedure, its risks and benefits, and alternative procedures
- The client giving consent has a right to have all questions answered satisfactorily

The nurse enters the room of a preoperative client to obtain the client's signature on the surgical consent form. Which question is most important for the nurse to ask the client?

A. When did the surgeon explain the procedure to you?
B. Is any member of your family going to be here during your surgery?
C. Have you been instructed in postoperative activities and restrictions?
D. Have you received any preoperative pain medication?

HESI Test Question Approach			
Positive?		YES	NO
Key Words			
Rephrase			
Rule Out Choices			
A	B	C	D

Death and Grief

- Stages of grief
  — Denial
  — Anger
  — Bargaining
  — Depression
  — Acceptance
- Encourage client to express anger
- *Do not* take away the defense mechanism/coping mechanism used in crisis
- How families deal with death/dying will vary by culture

Which assignment should the nurse delegate to a UAP in an acute care setting?

A. Hourly blood glucose checks for a client with a continuous insulin drip
B. Giving PO medications left at the bedside for the client to take after eating
C. Taking vital signs for an older client with left humerus and left tibial fractures
D. Replacing a client's decubitus dressing soiled from incontinence

HESI Test Question Approach			
Positive?		YES	NO
Key Words			
Rephrase			
Rule Out Choices			
A	B	C	D

Shock

Stages

- Stage 1: Initial
  — Early signs include *agitation*
  — Restlessness
  — Increased heart rate
  — Cool pale skin
- Stage 2: Compensatory
  — Cardiac output <4-6 L/min
  — BP systolic <100 mm Hg
  — Decreased urinary output
  — Confusion
  — Cerebral perfusion <70 mm Hg
- Stage 3: Progressive
  — Edema
  — Excessively low BP
  — Dysrhythmia
  — Weak thready pulses
- Stage 4: Irreversible
  — Profound hypotension
  — Unresponsive to vasopressors
  — Heart rate slows
  — Multiple organ failure
  — Severe hypoxemia

Types of Shock

- Hypovolemic
  — Most common
  — Related to internal or external blood/fluid loss
- Cardiogenic
  — Pump failure
  — Results in ↓ cardiac output
- Vasogenic
  — Failure of arteriolar resistance
  — Massive vasodilation and pooling of blood
- Septic
  — Endotoxins released from bacteria
  — Massive vasodilation and pooling

Treatment for Shock

- Replace blood volume or fluid loss
  — Lactated Ringers, albumin, whole blood, PRBCs
- Administer medications
  — Vasodilators
    • Nitroprusside (Nipride)
    • Hydralazine (Apresoline)
    • Labetalol hydrochloride (Normodyne, Trandate)
  — Vasoconstrictors
    • Dopamine (Dopram)
    • Dobutamine (Dobutrex)
    • Norepinephrine bitartrate (Levophed)
- Monitor
  — Vital signs
  — Mental status
  — Fluid status
  — Urine output

S — Solutions
H — Hemodynamic stability
O — Oxygen
C — Conserve heat
K — Keep feet up and head down
For cardiogenic shock and pulmonary edema - position patient to REDUCE venous return high Fowler's with legs down, ↓ workload on the heart, help to optimize the O_2 exchange

A client in shock develops a central venous pressure (CVP) of 2 cm of water and a mean arterial pressure (MAP) of 60 mm Hg. Which prescribed intervention should the nurse implement first?

A. Increase the rate of O_2 flow
B. Obtain arterial blood gas results
C. Insert an indwelling urinary catheter
D. Increase the rate of IV fluids

HESI Test Question Approach			
Positive?		YES	NO
Key Words			
Rephrase			
Rule Out Choices			
A	B	C	D

Septic shock is one component of the systemic inflammatory response syndrome (SIRS). The syndrome starts with an infection that progresses to *bacteremia*, then *sepsis*, then *severe sepsis*, then *septic shock*, and then multiple organ dysfunction syndrome (MODS).

Systemic Inflammatory Response Syndrome (SIRS) is a systemic inflammatory response to an assortment of insults, including sepsis, ischemia, infarction, and injury. Generalized inflammation in organs remote from the initial insult characterizes the syndrome.

Multiple Organ Dysfunction Syndrome (MODS) is the failure of two or more organ systems in an acutely ill patient such that homeostasis cannot be maintained without intervention. MODS results from SIRS. These two syndromes represent the ends of a continuum.

Nursing and collaborative management
■ The prognosis for the patient with MODS is poor.
■ The most common cause continues to be sepsis.
■ The most important goal is to prevent the progression of SIRS to MODS.
■ The nursing role is attentive assessment and ongoing monitoring to detect early signs of organ dysfunction.

Collaborative care focuses on:
■ Prevention and treatment of infection
■ Maintenance of tissue oxygenation
■ Nutritional and metabolic support
■ Support of individual failing organs

Disseminated Intravascular Coagulation (DIC)
■ DIC is an abnormal response of the normal clotting cascade stimulated by a disease process or disorder.
— DIC results from abnormally initiated and accelerated clotting.
— Subsequent decreases in clotting factors and platelets ensue.
— May lead to uncontrollable hemorrhage

11

- As more clots are made, more breakdown products from fibrinogen and fibrin are also formed. They work in three ways to interfere with blood coagulation.
  — Coat the platelets and interfere with platelet function
  — Interfere with thrombin and thereby disrupt coagulation
  — Attach to fibrinogen, which interferes with the process necessary to form a clot
- D-Dimer assay test measures the degree of fibrinolysis.
- Appropriate nursing interventions are essential to the survival of the client.
- Astute, ongoing assessment
  — Early detection of bleeding, both occult and overt, must be a primary goal.
  — The patient is assessed for signs of external and internal bleeding.
  — Active attention to manifestations of the syndrome
- Institution of appropriate treatment measures, which can be challenging and sometimes paradoxic
  — Heparin infusion

Acute Respiratory Distress Syndrome (ARDS)

- ARDS is considered to be present if the client has the following:
  — Refractory hypoxemia
  — Chest radiograph with new bilateral interstitial or alveolar infiltrates
  — The chest radiograph is often termed whiteout or white lung.
  — Pulmonary artery wedge pressure of 18 mm Hg or less and no evidence of heart failure
  — A predisposing condition for ARDS within 48 hours of clinical manifestations
- Alveolar capillary membrane damage with subsequent leakage of fluids into the interstitial spaces and the alveoli
- As ARDS progresses, it is associated with profound respiratory distress requiring endotracheal intubation and PPV.

Nursing Assessment

- Dyspnea
- Scattered crackles
- Intercostal retractions
- Pink frothy sputum
- Cyanosis
- Hypoxemia
- Hypercapnia
- Respiratory acidosis
- Impaired Gas Exchange ($\downarrow$ $\dot{V}/\dot{Q}$ perfusion ratio)
- Increased secretions
- Decreased cardiac output ($\downarrow$ venous return)

Nursing Plans and Interventions

- The overall goals for the patient with ARDS
  — Pao_2 of at least 60 mm Hg
  — Adequate lung ventilation to maintain normal pH

- The goals for a patient recovering from ARDS
  - Pao_2 within normal limits for age or baseline values on room air
  - Sao_2 greater than 90%
  - Patent airway
  - Clear lungs on auscultation
- Positive end-expiratory pressure (PEEP)
  - This ventilatory option creates positive pressure at end exhalation and restores functional residual capacity (FRC).

EMERGENCY, TERRORISM, AND DISASTER NURSING

Basic Life Support
- Cardiac arrest is the most common event requiring CPR

CPR and Choking Basics (Adults)
- Establish an airway
- Ventilate with two breaths
- Maintain circulation
- Perform CPR
- 30:2 ratio of compression/ventilation
- 100 compressions/min
- *Do not* try to intervene if choking person *can* speak, cough, or breathe

CPR and Choking Basics (Neonates and Children 1 to 8)
- Most common indications for CPR in children are *not* the same as for adults.
  - Neonates and infants: hypoxia, hypoglycemia, hypothermia, acidosis, hypercoagulability
  - Children: respiratory arrest, prolonged hypoxemia secondary to respiratory insult or shock, including septic shock
- Guidelines vary based on age of child.
  - Ventilation technique and rate
  - Compression technique and rate
  - How to manage the obstructed airway

Clinical Management
Communication Skills
- "Do it *my* way."
- Aggressive communication/authoritarian leader
- "Whatever … as long as you like me."
- Passive communication/laissez-faire leader
- "Let's consider the options available."
- Assertive communication/democratic leader

The charge nurse confronts a staff nurse whose behavior is resentful and negative after a change in unit policy is announced. The staff nurse states, "Don't blame me; nobody likes this idea." What is the charge nurse's priority action?

A. Confront the other staff members involved in the change of unit policy.
B. Call a unit meeting to review the reasons why the change was made.
C. Develop a written unit policy for the expression of complaints.
D. Encourage the nurse to be accountable for her own behavior.

HESI Test Question Approach			
Positive?		YES	NO
Key Words			
Rephrase			
Rule Out Choices			
A	B	C	D

Delegation Skills

Five rights of delegation
■ Right task
■ Right circumstance
■ Right person
■ Right direction/communication
■ Right supervision

The charge nurse is making assignments for each of four staff members, including a registered nurse (RN), a licensed practical nurse (LPN), and two UAPs. Which task is best to assign the LPN?

A. Maintain a 24-hour urine collection
B. Wean a client from a mechanical ventilator
C. Perform sterile wound irrigation
D. Obtain scheduled vital signs

HESI Test Question Approach			
Positive?		YES	NO
Key Words			
Rephrase			
Rule Out Choices			
A	B	C	D

Supervision Skills

■ Direction/guidance
■ Evaluation/monitoring
■ Follow-up

Which situation warrants a variance (incident) report by the nurse?

A. Refusal by a client to take prescribed medication
B. Improved status before completion of the course of medication
C. An allergic reaction to a prescribed medication
D. A client received medication prescribed for another client

HESI Test Question Approach			
Positive?		YES	NO
Key Words			
Rephrase			
Rule Out Choices			
A	B	C	D

DISASTER MANAGEMENT

- The nurse is an active member of teams in the event of biological, chemical, radioactive, mass trauma, and natural disasters.
- The nurse has a role at all three levels of disaster management.

Preparedness ... Response ... Recovery
- Levels of prevention in disaster management
  - Primary: planning, training, educating personnel and the public
  - Secondary: triage, treatment, shelter supervision
  - Tertiary: follow-up, recovery assistance, prevention of future disasters

Triage
- Goal: to maximize the number of survivors by sorting the injured as treatable and untreatable, using the criteria of potential for survival and availability of resources
- Color-coded system
- START (Simple Triage And Rapid Treatment) method
- Separate out walking wounded, move, evaluate later
- Three-step evaluation of others done one at a time
  - Respiration
  - Circulation
  - Mental status

BIOTERRORISM

- Review exposure information, assessment findings, and treatment for various agents:
  - Biological
  - Chemical
  - Radiation
- Questions may deal with disasters and bioterrorism as they affect the individual victim, families, and the community.

The nurse is completing discharge teaching for a group of postal employees who have been exposed to a powder form of anthrax. Which instruction has the highest priority?
A. Begin the prescribed antibiotics and continue for 60 days.
B. Watch for symptoms of anthrax for the next 7 days.
C. Make arrangements to be vaccinated for anthrax.
D. Explain to family members that anthrax is not contagious.

HESI Test Question Approach			
Positive?		YES	NO
Key Words			
Rephrase			
Rule Out Choices			
A	B	C	D

Preoperative Care

- Preoperative evaluation
  — Obtain a complete history including
  — List of current medications and allergies
  — Previous surgical experiences (response to anesthesia)
  — Signed consent
  — Ascertain that informed consent has been obtained before patient is sedated
- Preoperative teaching
  — NPO after midnight before surgery
  — Teach coughing and deep breathing, incentive spirometry
  — Review methods of pain control

Intraoperative Care

- Maintain client safety
- Provide psychosocial support
- Immediate postoperative care
  — Monitoring for signs and symptoms of shock
  — Position on side
  — Manage pain

Postoperative Care

Prevent common complications
- Urinary retention
  — Check for bladder distention
- Pulmonary problems
  — Check breath sounds
  — O_2 saturation
- Decreased peristalsis
  — Paralytic ileus
  — Absent bowel sounds
- Wound dehiscence
- Wound evisceration

3 Clinical Concepts and Mechanisms of Disease

PAIN

- Pain is whatever the client says it is.
- Pain occurs in all clinical settings.
- Nurses have a central role in pain assessment and management.
  - Assessing pain and communicating to other health care providers
  - Ensuring the initiation and coordination of adequate pain relief measures
  - Evaluating the effectiveness of interventions
  - Advocating for clients with pain
- Pain medications generally are divided into three categories.
  - Nonopioids for mild pain
  - Opioids for moderate to severe pain
  - Co-analgesic or adjuvant drugs for neuropathic pain

Types of Pain Medications
Nonopioid Analgesics

- Acetaminophen (Tylenol)
- Salicylates
  - Aspirin
  - Choline magnesium trisalicylate (Trilisate)
- Nonsteroidal antiinflammatory drugs (NSAIDs)
  - Ibuprofen (Motrin, Nuprin, Advil)
  - Indomethacin (Indocin)
  - Ketorolac (Toradol)
  - Diclofenac K (Cataflam)
- Cyclooxygenase-2 (COX-2) inhibitors
  - Celecoxib (Celebrex)

Opioid Analgesics

- Mu agonists
  - Morphine (Roxanol, MS Contin, Avinza, Kadian, Epimorph, MSIR, Oramorph SR)
  - Hydromorphone (Dilaudid)
  - Methadone (Dolophine)
  - Levorphanol (Levo-Dromoran)
  - Fentanyl (Sublimaze, Duragesic, Actiq)
  - Oxycodone (Percocet, Percodan, Endocet, Tylox, Roxicodone, OxyContin, Combunox)
  - Hydrocodone (Lortab, Vicodin, Zydone)
  - Codeine (Tylenol No. 3)
- Mixed agonist-antagonists
  - Pentazocine (Talwin)
  - Butorphanol (Stadol)

- Partial agonists
  — Buprenorphine (Buprenex)
  — Buprenorphine plus naloxone (Suboxone)
- Adjuvant drugs
  — Used for neuropathic pain

Nonpharmacological Pain Relief Techniques
- Noninvasive
  — Heat and cold application
  — Massage therapy
  — Relaxation techniques
  — Guided imagery
  — Biofeedback techniques
- Invasive
  — Nerve blocks
  — Interruption of neural pathways
  — Acupuncture

FLUIDS AND ELECTROLYTES

Fluid Volume Excess
- Causes
  — CHF (most common), renal failure, cirrhosis, over-hydration
- Symptoms
  — Peripheral edema, periorbital edema, elevated BP, dyspnea, altered LOC
- Lab findings
  — $\downarrow$ BUN, $\downarrow$ Hgb, $\downarrow$ Hct, $\downarrow$ serum osmolality, $\downarrow$ urine specific gravity
- Treatment
  — Diuretics, fluid restrictions, weigh daily, monitor K^+

Fluid Volume Deficit
- Causes
  — Inadequate fluid intake, hemorrhage, vomiting, diarrhea, massive edema
- Symptoms
  — Weight loss, oliguria, postural hypotension
- Lab findings
  — BUN and creatinine, $\uparrow$ Hgb, $\uparrow$ Hct, $\uparrow$ urine specific gravity
- Treatment
  — Strict I & O, replace with isotonic fluids, monitor BP, weigh daily

Electrolyte Balance
- Intracellular
  — K^+ maintains osmotic pressure.
  — K^+ imbalances are potentially life threatening.
- Extracellular
  — Na^+ maintains most abundant osmotic pressure.
- When there is either ECF or ICF change in concentration, remember that fluid shifts from the area of *lesser* concentration to the area of *greater* concentration.

Hyponatremia
- Na^+ <135 mEq/L
- Muscle cramps, confusion
- Check BP frequently
- Restrict fluids, cautious IV replacement as needed

18

Hypernatremia

- Na^+ >145 mEq/L
- Pulmonary edema, seizures, thirst, fever
- No IVs that contain sodium
- Restrict sodium in diet
- Weigh daily

Hypokalemia

- K^+ <3.5 mEq/L
- Rapid, thready pulse, flat T waves, fatigue, anorexia, muscle cramps
- IV potassium supplements
- Encourage foods high in K^+ (bananas, oranges, spinach)

Hyperkalemia

- K^+ >5.0 mEq/L
- Tall tented T waves, bradycardia, muscle weakness
- 10%-20% glucose with regular insulin
- Kayexalate
- Renal dialysis may be required

Hypocalcemia

- Ca^{++} <8.5 mEq/L
- + Trousseau's sign, + Chvostek's sign, diarrhea, numbness, convulsions
- Administer calcium supplements
- IV calcium give slowly
- Increase dietary calcium

Hypercalcemia

- Ca^{++} >10.5 mEq/L
- Muscle weakness, constipation, nausea and vomiting (N/V), dysrhythmias, behavioral changes
- Limit vitamin D intake
- Avoid calcium-based antacids
- Calcitonin to reduce calcium
- Renal dialysis may be required

IV Therapy

Types of IV fluids

- Isotonic: 0.9% NS, LR, D_5W
- Hypotonic: 0.5% NS, 0.45% NS
- Hypertonic: D_5 0.45% NS, D_5LR, D_5NS

ACID BASE

Basics for NCLEX-RN Interpret ABG results

- pH
  — Normal 7.35 to 7.45
  — <7.35 = acidosis
  — >7.45 = alkalosis
- P_{CO_2}
  — Normal 35 to 45 mm Hg
  — >45 = acidosis
  — <35 = alkalosis
- HCO_3^-
  — Normal 22 to 26 mEq/L
  — <22 = acidosis
  — >26 = alkalosis

INFECTION AND HIV

Infection

- Invasion of the body by a pathogen
- Response to the invasion
  — Localized
  — Systemic
- Nosocomial infections
  — Acquired as a result of exposure to a microorganism in a hospital setting

Human Immunodeficiency Virus

Routes of Transmission

- Unprotected sexual contact
  — Most common mode of transmission
- Exposure to blood through drug-using equipment
- Perinatal transmission
  — Most common route of infection for children
  — Can occur during pregnancy, at the time of delivery, or after birth through breast-feeding

Symptoms

- May begin with flulike symptoms in the earliest stage and advance to …
  — Severe weight loss
  — Secondary infections
  — Cancers
  — Neurological disease

HIV Collaborative Management

- Monitoring HIV disease progression and immune function
- Initiating and monitoring antiretroviral therapy (ART)
- Preventing the development of opportunistic diseases
- Detecting and treating opportunistic diseases
- Managing symptoms
- Preventing or decreasing the complications of treatment
- Preventing further transmission of HIV
  — Ongoing assessment, interactions with the client, and client education and support are required to accomplish these objectives.

HIV Drug Therapy

The goals of drug therapy:

- Decrease the viral load
- Maintain or raise $CD4^+$ T-cell counts
- Delay the development of HIV-related symptoms and opportunistic diseases

HIV Medications

- Nucleoside reverse transcriptase inhibitors (NRTIs)
  — Zidovudine (AZT, ZDV, Retrovir)
  — Lamivudine (3TC, Epivir)
  — Abacavir (Ziagen)
  — Emtricitabine (FTC, Emtriva)
- Nucleotide reverse transcriptase inhibitor (NtRTI)
  — Tenofovir DF (Viread)
- Nonnucleoside reverse transcriptase inhibitors (NNRTIs)
- Enzymes, hepatotoxicity
  — Nevirapine (Viramune)

— Delavirdine (Rescriptor)
— Efavirenz (Sustiva)
- Protease inhibitors (PIs)
— Indinavir (Crixivan)
— Ritonavir (Norvir)
— Nelfinavir (Viracept)
— Amprenavir (Agenerase)
— Atazanavir (Reyataz)
— Fosamprenavir (Lexiva)
— Tipranavir (Aptivus)
— Darunavir (Prezista)
- Entry inhibitor
— Enfuvirtide (Fuzeon)

Pediatric HIV
- Common clinical manifestations of HIV infection in children
- Lymphadenopathy
- Hepatosplenomegaly
- Oral candidiasis
- Chronic or recurrent diarrhea
- Failure to thrive
- Developmental delay
- Parotitis

Considerations
- Education concerns transmission and control of infectious diseases.
- Safety issues include appropriate storage of special medications and equipment.
- Prevention is a key component of HIV education.
- Aggressive pain management is essential.
- Common psychosocial concerns include disclosure of the diagnosis.

Evaluation
- For children 18 months of age and older
— HIV enzyme-linked immunosorbent assay (ELISA)
— Western blot immunoassay
- For infants younger than 18 months
— HIV polymerase chain reaction (PCR)
— In infants born to HIV-infected mothers, these assays will be positive because of the presence of maternal antibodies derived transplacentally.

CANCER

Leukemia
- Acute myelogenous leukemia (AML)
— Inability of leukocytes to mature; those that do are abnormal
— 60-70 years old
- Chronic myelogenous leukemia (CML)
— Abnormal production of granulocytic cells
— 20-60 years of age (peak around 45 years)
- Acute lymphocytic leukemia (ALL)
— Abnormal leukocytes in blood-forming tissue
— Before 14 years of age and older adults
- Chronic lymphocytic leukemia (CLL)
— Increased production of leukocytes and lymphocytes within the bone marrow, spleen, and liver
— 50-70 years of age

[handwritten note: Overgrowth of immature WBCs]

Nursing Assessment

- General
  — Fever, generalized lymphadenopathy, lethargy
- Integumentary
  — Pallor or jaundice; petechiae, ecchymoses, purpura, reddish brown to purple cutaneous infiltrates, macules, and papules
- Cardiovascular
  — Tachycardia, systolic murmurs
- Gastrointestinal
  — Gingival bleeding and hyperplasia; oral ulcerations, herpes, and *Candida* infections; perirectal irritation and infection; hepatomegaly, splenomegaly
- Neurological
  — Seizures, disorientation, confusion, decreased coordination, cranial nerve palsies, papilledema
- Musculoskeletal
  — Muscle wasting, bone pain, joint pain

Medications for Leukemia

- Alkylating agents
- Antimetabolites
- Corticosteroids
- Nitrosoureas
- Mitotic inhibitors/vinca alkaloids
- Biological/targeted therapy
- Podophyllotoxin
- Retinoid

Nursing Interventions for Clients with Immunodeficiency and/or Bone Marrow Suppression

- Monitor WBC count
- Report fever or S/S of infection to physician as soon as symptoms are recognized
- Teach infection control measures
- Administer IV antibiotics as ordered:
  — Trough (draw shortly before administration)
  — Peak (30 minutes to 1 hour after administration)

Hodgkin's Lymphoma
Etiology

- Epstein-Barr virus (EBV), genetic predisposition, and exposure to occupational toxins

Diagnosis

- The main diagnostic feature of Hodgkin's lymphoma is the presence of Reed-Sternberg cells in lymph node biopsy specimens.

Nursing Assessment

- Weight loss
- Fatigue
- Weakness
- Chills, fever, night sweats
- Tachycardia

Nursing Interventions

- Non-Hodgkin's chemotherapy
- Radiation therapy
- Pain management due to tumors
- Pancytopenia
- Fertility
- Secondary malignancies

Non-Hodgkin's Lymphoma

Etiology

- Immunosuppressant medications, age and HIV, Epstein-Barr virus (EBV)
- Affects the beta or T cells

Diagnosis

- Same as for Hodgkin's lymphoma
- MRI, CT scan, and barium enemas

Nursing Assessment

- Painless lymph node enlargement (lymphadenopathy)
- Depending on where the disease has spread
- Same as Hodgkin's lymphoma

Nursing Interventions

- Chemotherapy (sometimes radiation therapy)
- Monoclonal antibodies
- Symptom management (depending on affected system)

Nursing Plans and Interventions

- Strict aseptic technique
- Protect client from infection
- Monitor for S/S of anemia
- High-nutrient diet
- Emotional support to client and family
- Treatment needs to be completed to help ensure survival
- Highly curable disease when diagnosed early and treatment is completed

A client is receiving vancomycin (Vancocin) IV and has a prescription for peak and trough levels. Before administering the next dose, what action should the nurse implement?
A. Verify the culture and sensitivity results.
B. Review the client's WBC count.
C. Schedule the collection of blood for a peak level.
D. Determine if the trough level has been collected.

Administration of Chemotherapeutic Agents

- Strict guidelines must be followed!
- Normally administered by chemotherapy-certified RN
- Pregnant nurses should not administer most of these agents
- Wear gloves when handling drugs

HESI Test Question Approach			
Positive?		YES	NO
Key Words			
Rephrase			
Rule Out Choices			
A	B	C	D

- Types of IV catheters
  — Hickman
  — Broviac
  — Port-a-cath

A client who is receiving chemotherapy has a CBC result showing a hemoglobin of 8.5 g/dL, hematocrit of 32%, and WBC count of 6500 cells/mm³. Which meal choice is best?
A. Grilled chicken, rice, fresh fruit salad, milk
B. Broiled steak, whole wheat rolls, spinach salad, coffee
C. Smoked ham, mashed potatoes, applesauce, iced tea
D. Tuna noodle casserole, garden salad, lemonade

HESI Test Question Approach		
Positive?	YES	NO
Key Words		
Rephrase		
Rule Out Choices		
A	B	C	D

Head and Neck Cancer

- Typically squamous cell in origin.
- Tumor sites
  — Paranasal sinuses
  — Oral cavity
  — Nasopharynx
  — Oropharynx
  — Larynx
- Disability is great because of the potential loss of voice, disfigurement, and social consequences.
- Head and neck cancer is most common in males over the age of 50 and is related to heavy tobacco and alcohol intake.

Lung Cancer

- Number one cancer in the United States!
- The increase in death rates for both men and women is directly related to cigarette smoking.

Nursing Assessment

- Symptoms of lung cancer are not usually apparent until the disease is in the advanced stages.
- Persistent hacking cough may be either dry or productive with blood-tinged sputum.
- Hoarseness
- Dyspnea
- Abnormal chest radiograph
- Positive sputum on cytological examination

Treatment

- Chemotherapy
- Radiation therapy
- Surgical intervention
  — Pneumonectomy removal of entire lung
  — Lobectomy segmental resection
- Nursing care depends upon the type of medical treatment prescribed.

Immediate Postoperative Care

- Promoting ventilation and reexpansion of the lung by:
  — Maintaining a clear airway
  — Maintaining the closed drainage system if one is used
- Promoting arm exercises to maintain full use on the operated side
- Promoting nutrition
  — Monitoring the incision for bleeding and subcutaneous emphysema

Colorectal Cancer

- The third most common form of cancer and the second leading cause of cancer-related deaths in the United States
  — Adenocarcinoma most common
  — Common metastasis to the liver

Symptoms

- Rectal bleeding
- Change in bowel habits
- Abdominal pain, weight loss, N/V
- Ribbonlike stool
- Sensation of incomplete evacuation

Diagnostic Testing

- Testing of stool for occult blood
- Colonoscopy

Treatment Modalities

- Chemotherapy
- Radiation therapy
- Adjunctive or palliative

Surgical Intervention

- Bowel resection
- Temporary colostomy
- Permanent colostomy

Postoperative Care Issues

- Stoma care
  — Loop
  — Double-barrel
  — End stoma
- Incision care
  — Abdominal
  — Perineal
- Packing and drains
  — HemoVac
  — Jackson-Pratt

Stoma Assessment

- The stoma should be pink.
- There is mild to moderate swelling of the stoma the first 2 to 3 weeks after surgery.
- The pouching system
  — Skin barrier
  — Bag or pouch
  — Adhesive

- Help clients cope with the stoma
  — Provide information
  — Teach practical stoma care techniques
  — Help clients address issues surrounding social interactions
    • Employment
    • Body image
    • Sexuality

The nurse is caring for a client who is 24-hours post-procedure for a hemicolectomy with a temporary colostomy placement. The assessment finds that the client's stoma is dry and dark red. What action should the nurse implement based on this finding?
A. Notify the healthcare provider of the finding
B. Document the finding in the client's record
C. Replace the pouch system over the stoma
D. Place petrolatum gauze dressing on stoma

HESI Test Question Approach				
Positive?			YES	NO
Key Words				
Rephrase				
Rule Out Choices				
A		B	C	D

Breast Cancer
- Risks
  — Family history
  — Age
  — Hyperestrogenism
  — Radiation exposure
- A great majority are discovered through breast self-examination
- Tumors tend to be in upper outer quadrant
  — Ductal carcinoma
  — Lobar carcinoma
  — Ductal carcinoma in situ
  — Inflammatory breast cancer (most aggressive)
  — Paget's disease (areola and nipple)
- Recommend mammogram every 1 to 2 years after age 40, then annual mammograms after age 50

Treatment Modalities
- Surgical
  — Mastectomy
  — Modified radical mastectomy
  — Lumpectomy
  — Tissue expansion and breast implants
  — Musculocutaneous flap procedure
- Radiation
- Chemotherapy
- Hormonal therapy
  — Tamoxifen (Nolvadex) blocks estrogen receptors
  — Fulvestrant (Faslodex) destroys estrogen receptors
  — Anastrozole (Arimidex), letrozole (Femara) prevents production of estrogen
- Biological targeted therapies
- Monoclonal antibodies

Nursing Assessment
- Hard lump not freely moveable
- Dimpling in skin
- Change in skin color
- Confirmed on mammogram and biopsy with frozen sections

Nursing Interventions
- Preoperative
  — Assess expectations
- Postoperative
  — Monitor for bleeding
  — Position arm on operative side on a pillow
  — No BP, IVs, or injections on operative side
  — Provide emotional support, recognize the grieving process

Cancer of the Cervix
- A human papillomavirus (HPV) is a virus that infects the skin and mucous membranes of humans.
- Vaccine approved for females ages 9 to 26 (also protects vaccinated females and males, ages 9 to 26, against 90% genital warts cases)
- Requires three shots over 6 months
- Trade names for HPV vaccines: Gardasil and Cervarix
- Usually detected early with a Pap test
- Dysplasia treated with cryosurgery, laser, conization, possibly hysterectomy
- Early carcinoma treated with hysterectomy or intra-cavity radiation
- Late carcinoma treated with radiation, chemotherapy, and/or pelvic exenteration

Care of the Client with Radiation Implants
- Client is *not* radioactive
- Implants do contain radioactivity
- Place in private room
- No pregnant caretakers or pregnant visitors
- Keep lead-lined container in the room
- All client secretions can be potentially radioactive
- Wear radiation badge when providing care

Ovarian Cancer
- Greatest risk factor is family history
- Asymptomatic in early stages
- Generalized feeling of abdominal fullness
- Sense of pelvic heaviness
- Loss of appetite
- Change in bowel habit
- Late stage symptoms
- Pelvic discomfort
- Low back pain
- Abdominal pain
- Ovarian cancer is the leading cause of death from gynecological cancers

Testicular Cancer

- Feeling of heaviness in lower abdomen
- Painless lump/swelling
- Postoperative orchiectomy
- Observe for bleeding
- Encourage genetic counseling (sperm banking)
- Postoperative management
  — Monitor for urine leaks
  — Avoid rectal manipulation
  — Low residue diet

Cancer of the Prostate

- Symptoms of urinary obstruction
- Elevated prostate-specific antigen (PSA)
- Surgical removal of the prostate
- Follow-up radiation and chemotherapy

The charge nurse is assigning rooms for four new clients, but only one private room is available on the oncology unit. Which client should be placed in the private room? The client with
A. Ovarian cancer receiving chemotherapy
B. Breast cancer receiving external beam radiation
C. Prostate cancer following transurethral resection
D. Cervical cancer with intracavity radiation

HESI Test Question Approach		
Positive?	YES	NO
Key Words		
Rephrase		
Rule Out Choices		
A	B	C	D

Brain Tumor

- Primary malignant tumors can arise in any area of brain tissue
- Benign tumors can continue to grow and cause problems with ↑ICP
- Assess for headache, vomiting, seizures, aphasia, abnormal CT, MRI, or PET scan

Nursing Plans and Interventions

- Similar to head injury client
- Major concern is ↑ ICP
- Keep HOB elevated 30 to 40 degrees
- Radiation therapy
- Chemotherapy
- Surgical removal: Craniotomy
- Postoperative care
  — Monitor for ↑ICP
  — CSF leakage
  — Monitor respiratory status closely
  — Monitor for seizure activity

4 Oxygenation, Ventilation, Transportation, and Perfusion

A male client who is 1-day postoperative after a left pneumonectomy is lying on his right side with the head of bed (HOB) elevated 10 degrees. The nurse assesses his respiratory rate at 32 breaths/min. What action should the nurse implement first?

A. Elevate the head of the bed
B. Assist to supine position
C. Measure O_2 saturation
D. Administer PRN morphine IV

HESI Test Question Approach			
Positive?		YES	NO
Key Words			
Rephrase			
Rule Out Choices			
A	B	C	D

Pneumonia Pathophysiology

Pneumonia results in inflammation of lung tissue causing consolidation of exudate.

- *Pathogens*
  — Bacterial (gram-negative most severe), viral (rare), fungal
- Host's physical status
- Aspiration
- Inhalation
- Hypostatic
- Anatomical areas
- Lung parenchyma
- Pleurae

The spouse of a 94-year-old reports to the home health nurse that his wife has become increasingly confused over the last few days and has developed a cough. Which assessment should the nurse perform first?

A. Jugular vein distention
B. Skin turgor
C. Oxygen saturation
D. Pupillary response to light

HESI Test Question Approach			
Positive?		YES	NO
Key Words			
Rephrase			
Rule Out Choices			
A	B	C	D

Nursing Assessment

- Tachypnea
- Fever abrupt onset
- Dyspnea
- Cyanosis
- Mental status changes
- Crackles, decreased breath sounds
- Dullness with percussion

Nursing Plans and Interventions

- Hand washing to reduce cross contamination
- Antibiotics
- Isolation if prescribed
- Administer fluids
- Manage pain
- Monitor oxygenation (humidified to loosen secretions)

Chronic Airflow Limitation (CAL)

- Asthma—reversible disease
- Chronic obstructive pulmonary disease (COPD)—chronic progressive disease
- Emphysema
- Chronic bronchitis

Chronic Bronchitis

- Pathophysiology
- Chronic sputum with cough production on a daily basis for a minimum of 3 mo/yr
- Chronic hypoxemia/cor pulmonale
- Increase in mucus, cilia production
- Increase in bronchial wall thickness (obstructs air flow)
- Exacerbations usually due to infection
- Increased $\dot{V}/\dot{Q}$ abnormalities
- Increased CO_2 retention/acidemia
- Increased pulmonary artery pressure (PAP) = cor pulmonale
- Reduced responsiveness of respiratory center to hypoxemic stimuli

Emphysema

- Abnormal enlargement of the air spaces distal to the terminal alveolar walls
- Increased dyspnea/work of breathing
  — Reduced gas exchange surface area
  — Increased air trapping (increased anterior-posterior diameter)
  — Decreased capillary network
  — Increased work/increased O_2 consumption

COPD Assessment Data

- Inspection
  — Bronchitis
    - *Right-sided heart failure*
    - *Cyanosis distended neck veins*
  — Emphysema
    - *Pursed-lip breathing*
    - *Noncyanotic, thin*
- Auscultation
  — Bronchitis
    - *Crackles*

Antiinfective Medications

- Penicillins
  — Semisynthetic penicillins
    - Oxacillin (Bactoill)
  — Antipseudomonal penicillins
    - Piperacillin (Pipracil)
- Tetracyclines
  — Doxycycline hyclate (Vibramycin)
- Aminoglycosides
  — Gentamicin sulfate (Garamycin)
- Cephalosporins
  — Ceftriaxone (Rocephin)
- Macrolides
  — Clarithromycin (Biaxin)
- Fluoroquinolones
  — Ciprofloxacin (Cipro)

COPD Etiology/Precipitating Factors

- Cigarette smoking
- Environmental/occupational exposure
- Genetic predisposition

- *Rhonchi*
- *Expiratory wheezes*
— Emphysema
  - *Distant breath sounds*
  - *Quiet breath sounds*
  - *Wheezes*

COPD Nursing Plans and Interventions

- Lowest O_2 to prevent CO_2 retention
  — Respiratory drive based on O_2 levels
- Monitor for signs and symptoms (S/S) of fluid overload
- Baseline ABGs for CO_2 retainers
- Client teaching pursed-lip breathing
- Orthopneic position

Reactive Airway Disease

Asthma

- Inflammatory disorder of the airways that is characterized by an exaggerated bronchoconstrictor response to a wide variety of stimuli
- Allergens
- Environmental irritants
- Cold air
- Exercise
- Beta-blockers
- Respiratory infection
- Emotional stress
- Reflux esophagitis

Drug Therapy for Asthma and COPD

β_2-Adrenergic Agonists
- Inhaled: Short-Acting
  — Metaproterenol (Alupent, Metaprel) nebulizer, oral tablets, elixir, MDI (metered-dose inhaler)
  — Albuterol (Proventil, Proventil, Ventolin HFA, Salbutamol, Volmax) nebulizer, MDI, oral tablets, Rotahaler
  — Levalbuterol (Xopenex, Xopenex HFA) nebulizer, MDI
  — Pirbuterol (Maxair) MDI
  — Terbutaline (Bricanyl, Brethine) Oral tablets, nebulizer, subcutaneous, MDI
  — Bitolterol (Tornalate) MDI, nebulizer
- Inhaled: long-acting
  — Salmeterol (Serevent) DPI (dry powder inhaler)
  — Formoterol (Foradil) DPI
- Immediate-acting
  — Epinephrine (Adrenalin) subcutaneous
- Corticosteroids
  — Hydrocortisone (Solu-Cortef) IV
  — Methylprednisolone (Medrol, Solu-Medrol) oral
  — Prednisone IV
  — Beclomethasone (Vanceril, Beclovent, Vanceril DS, Qvar, Qvar HFA) oral
  — Triamcinolone (Azmacort)
  — Flunisolide (AeroBid, AeroBid-M)
  — Fluticasone (Flovent HFA, Flovent Diskus)
  — Budesonide (Pulmicort Turbuhaler, Pulmicort Respules)
  — Mometasone (Asmanex Twisthaler)

Bronchodilators

- Long-acting inhaled β_2-adrenergic agonists
- Long-acting oral β_2-adrenergic agonists
- Theophylline
- Short-acting inhaled β_2-adrenergic agonists
- Anticholinergics (inhaled)

- Anticholinergics
  — Short-acting ipratropium (Atrovent) Nebulizer, MDI
  — Long-Acting tiotropium (Spiriva) DPI
- Leukotriene modifiers
  — Leukotriene receptor blocker zafirlukast (Accolate) oral tablets
  — Leukotriene inhibitor zileuton (Zyflo) oral tablets
- Mast cell stabilizers
  — Cromolyn (Intal) nebulizer, MDI
  — Nedocromil (Tilade) MDI
- IgE antagonist omalizumab (Xolair) Subcutaneous injection
- Leukotriene modifiers
  — Leukotriene receptor blocker
    Zafirlukast (Accolate) oral tablets Montelukast (Singulair) oral tablets, chewable tablets, oral granules
  — Leukotriene inhibitor zileuton (Zyflo) oral tablets
- Methylxanthines
  — IV agent: Aminophylline (rarely used) oral tablets, IV, elixir, sustained-release tablets
  — Oral: Elixophyllin, Quibron, Slo-bid, Theochron, Theolair, Theo-24, Uniphyl
- Combination Agents
  — Ipratropium and albuterol (Combivent, DuoNeb) MDI, nebulizer
  — Fluticasone/salmeterol (Advair) DPI
  — Budesonide/formoterol (Symbicort) MDI

Nursing Assessment

- Dyspnea, wheezing, chest tightness
- Assess precipitating factors
- Medication history

Nursing Interventions

- Monitor respirations and assess breath sounds
- Monitor oxygen saturation
- Monitor mental status
- Chest physiotherapy
- Assess peripheral pulses and warmth and color of extremities
- Position for maximum ventilation
- Encourage slow, pursed-lip breathing.
- Encourage abdominal breathing
- Administer humidified oxygen therapy

The nurse palpates a crackling sensation of the skin around the chest tube insertion site of a client after thoracic surgery. What action should the nurse implement?
A. Return to surgery
B. Prepare for insertion of a larger chest tube
C. Increase the water seal suction pressure
D. Continue to monitor

HESI Test Question Approach			
Positive?		YES	NO
Key Words			
Rephrase			
Rule Out Choices			
A	B	C	D

Tuberculosis (TB)

TB is an infectious disease caused by the bacillus *Mycobacterium tuberculosis* or the tubercle bacillus, an acid-fast organism.

Resurgence of TB in the United States
- Related to HIV infection
- Multidrug-resistant TB (MDR-TB)
  — Rifampin
  — Isoniazid
- Seen disproportionately in poor, underserved, and minorities

Nursing Assessment
- Low-grade fever
- Pallor
- Chills
- Night sweats
- Easy fatigability
- Anorexia
- Weight loss

Nursing Interventions
- Respiratory isolation
- Medication regimen
  — Isoniazid (INH therapy)
  — Pyridoxine (vitamin B_6)
  — Rifampin (Rifadin)
  — Pyrazinamide
  — Take as prescribed for 9 to 12 months
  — Teach side effects

TB Drugs
First-Line Drugs
(Bacteriocidal against rapidly dividing cells and/or against semidormant bacteria)
- Isoniazid (INH): clinical hepatitis, fulminant hepatitis, peripheral neurotoxicity
- Rifampin (Rifadin): cutaneous reactions, GI disturbance (nausea, anorexia, abdominal pain), flulike syndrome, hepatotoxicity, immunological reactions, orange discoloration of bodily fluids (sputum, urine, sweat, tears)
- Ethambutol (Myambutol): retrobulbar neuritis (decreased red-green color discrimination), skin rash
- Rifabutin (Mycobutin): hematologic toxicity, GI symptoms, polyarthralgias, pseudojaundice, orange discoloration of bodily fluids
- Pyrazinamide (PZA): hepatotoxicity, GI symptoms (nausea, vomiting), polyarthralgias, skin rash, hyperuricemia, dermatitis
- Rifapentine (Priftin)

Tuberculosis
Second-Line Drugs: Bacteriocidal and/or Bacteriostatic and/or inhibits cell wall synthesis

cycloserine (Seromycin)
- Central nervous system effects (headache, restless, seizures, psychosis): given with pyridoxine to prevent neurotoxic effects

ethionamide (Trecator)
- Hepatotoxicity, neurotoxicity, GI effects (metallic taste, nausea, vomiting), endocrine effects (hypothyroid, impotence)

streptomycin
- Ototoxicity, neurotoxicity, nephrotoxicity

capreomycin (Capastat)
- Ototoxicity, nephrotoxicity

kanamycin (Kantrex) and amikacin
- Ototoxicity, nephrotoxicity

para-aminosalicylic acid (PAS)
- Hepatotoxicity, GI distress, malabsorption syndrome, coagulopathy

Fluoroquinolones: levofloxacin (Levaquin), moxifloxacin (Avelox, Vigamox), gatifloxacin (Tequin)
- GI disturbance, neurologic effects (dizzy, headache), rash

Hematologic Problems
Anemia
- Decreased erythrocyte production
- Decreased hemoglobin synthesis
  — Iron deficiency anemia
  — Thalassemias (decreased globin synthesis)
  — Sideroblastic anemia (decreased porphyrin)
- Defective DNA synthesis
  — Cobalamin (vitamin B_{12}) deficiency
  — Folic acid deficiency
- Decreased number of erythrocyte precursors
  — Aplastic anemia
- Anemia of myeloproliferative diseases (e.g., leukemia) and myelodysplasia
- Chronic diseases or disorders
- Chemotherapy
- Blood loss
  — Acute
  — Trauma
- Blood vessel rupture
- Chronic gastritis
- Menstrual flow
- Hemorrhoids
- Increased erythrocyte destruction

Nursing Assessment
- Pallor
- Fatigue
- Exercise intolerance
- Tachycardia
- Dyspnea
- Assess for risk factors
- Diet low in iron, vitamin B_{12} deficiency, history of bleeding, medications taken
- Hgb <10, Hct <36, RBC <4

Blood Transfusions
Blood Groups and Types
- The ABO system includes A, B, O, and AB blood types.
- Rh factor is an antigenic substance in the erythrocytes.
- If blood is mismatched during transfusion, a transfusion reaction occurs.
  — The transfusion reaction is an antigen-antibody reaction.
  — It can range from a mild response to severe anaphylactic shock.

Types of Blood Products
- Red blood cells (RBCs)
  — Packed RBCs (PRBCs)
  — Autologous PRBCs
  — Washed RBCs
  — Frozen RBCs
  — Leukocyte-poor RBCs
  — RBC units with high number of reticulocytes (young RBCs)
- Other cellular components
  — Platelets
  — Granulocytes

Intrinsic Causes
- Abnormal hemoglobin (HbS–sickle cell anemia)
- Enzyme deficiency (G6PD)
- Membrane abnormalities (paroxysmal nocturnal hemoglobinuria, hereditary spherocytosis)

Extrinsic Causes
- Physical trauma (prosthetic heart valves, extracorporeal circulation)
- Antibodies (isoimmune and autoimmune)
- Infectious agents, medications, and toxins

Nursing Interventions
- Treatment of underlying pathology
- Administer blood products as ordered
- Diet should be high in iron-rich foods, folic acid, vitamin B_{12}, vitamin B_6, amino acids, and vitamin C
  — Parenteral iron is given using Z-track technique

Types of Reactions
- Acute hemolytic
- Febrile, nonhemolytic (most common)
- Mild allergic
- Anaphylactic
- Delayed hemolytic

- Plasma components
  — Fresh frozen plasma (FFP)
  — Cryoprecipitate
  — Serum albumin
  — Plasma protein fraction (PPF)
  — Immune serum globulin

Nursing Interventions
- Assessment before, during, and after the transfusion including the IV site
- Confirm informed consent
- Identify the compatibility
- Initiation of a transfusion slowly then maintain the infusion rate
  — 1 unit of packed RBCs is transfused in 2 to 4 hours.

A client who is receiving a transfusion of packed red blood cells has an inflamed IV site. What action should the nurse implement?
A. Double-check the blood type of the unit of blood transfusing with another nurse.
B. Discontinue the transfusion and send the remaining blood and tubing to the lab.
C. Immediately start a new IV at another site and resume the transfusion at the new site.
D. Continue to monitor the site for signs of infection and notify the healthcare provider.

Hypertension (HTN)
- Persistent BP elevation >140/90mm Hg
- Risk factors:
  — Nonmodifiable: family history, gender, age, ethnicity
  — Modifiable: use of alcohol, tobacco, caffeine; sedentary lifestyle; obesity

Medications:
- Diuretics
  — HCTZ
- ACE inhibitors
  — lisinopril (Zestril)
- Calcium channel blockers
  — verapamil (Isoptin)
- Beta blockers
  — metoprolol (Lopressor)
- ARBs
  — valsartan (Diovan)
- Centrally-acting
  — clonidine (Catapres)

Coronary Artery Disease (CAD)
- Prevalent etiologies of CAD
  — Atherosclerosis: Partially or completely blocked coronary arteries
  — Coronary vasospasm
  — Microvascular angina
- CAD results in ischemia and infarction of myocardial tissue

HESI Test Question Approach		
Positive?	YES	NO
Key Words		
Rephrase		
Rule Out Choices		
A	B	C	D

HTN Education
Number one cause of stroke (cerebrovascular accident, CVA) is noncompliance with HTN medications

35

- LAD (left anterior descending artery) most commonly affected
- CAD remains the number one health problem in the United States

Heart Failure
Etiology
- Coronary artery disease (CAD), prior MI
- Chronic HTN
- Cardiomyopathy
  — Dilated
- Idiopathic
- Thyroid
- Diabetes
  — Restrictive
  — Ischemic
- Valvular and congenital heart disease
- Pulmonary diseases

Left-Sided Heart Failure (LHF)
- Causes: LV infarct, cardiomyopathy
- Symptoms: dyspnea, cough, fluid accumulation in lungs
- Signs: S3 gallop, tachycardia, inspiratory rales beginning at lung bases, expiratory wheezes due to bronchospasms (misdiagnosed with asthma)
- Laboratory findings: ABGs reveal hypoxemia, chest radiograph shows pulmonary edema or pleural effusions

Right-Sided Heart Failure (RHF) Systemic Congestion
- Causes: LHF, RV infarct, pulmonary or tricuspid valve disease, pulmonary HTN, COPD, PE
- Symptoms: dyspnea on exertion, fatigue, weight gain, fluid retention
- Signs: increased central venous pressure (CVP), jugular venous distention (JVD) >3-4 cm, hepatomegaly, ascites, peripheral or sacral edema, pleural and pericardial effusions are also not uncommon

Sodium and Volume Homeostasis
- As CO decreases, renal perfusion decreases.
- This activates the renin-angiotensin system.
- This causes fluid retention.

Pharmacological Management
- Angiotensin-converting enzyme (ACE) inhibitors
  — Captopril
  — Enalapril
  — Fosinopril
  — Lisinopril
  — Quinapril
  — Ramipril
  — Perindopril
  — Benazepril
- Diuretics
- Loop diuretics
  — Furosemide
  — Bumetanide
  — Torsemide

RHF Laboratory Tests
- Liver function shows hepatic congestion
- Increased liver enzymes, increased PT, INR
- Hyponatremia (fluid restriction only if Na^+ <132 mg/dL
- Increased BUN/creatinine = decreased renal perfusion

- Thiazides
  — Thiazide-related drug: metolazone
- Aldosterone antagonists
  — Spironolactone
  — Eplerenone
- Inotropes
  — Digoxin
  — Dobutamine
- Phosphodiesterase inhibitors
  — Milrinone
- Natriuretic peptides
  — Nesiritide
- Beta-blockers
  — Metoprolol
  — Carvedilol
  — Bisoprolol
- Angiotensin II receptor blockers
  — Losartan
  — Candesartan
  — Valsartan
- Vasodilators
  — Nitrates: isosorbide dinitrate
  — Hydralazine
  — Nitroprusside
  — Prazosin
- Dopamine agonist
  — Dopamine
- Analgesics
  — Morphine sulfate
- Anticoagulants
  — Warfarin
  — Aspirin

Nursing Management

- Activity
  — Regular exercise strongly encouraged—improves function of skeletal muscle more than changes in myocardial function
- Diet
  — Limit sodium intake
  — Fluid restriction only if Na^+ <132 mg/dL
  — Avoid excessive fluids
  — Avoid alcohol—depresses myocardial contractility
  — If CAD, low cholesterol, low fat, low Na^+

The nurse is administering 0900 medications to three clients on a telemetry unit when the unlicensed assistive personnel (UAP) reports that another client is complaining of a sudden onset of substernal discomfort. What action should the nurse implement?

A. Ask the UAP to obtain the client's VS
B. Assess the client's discomfort
C. Advise the client to rest in bed
D. Observe the client's ECG pattern

HESI Test Question Approach			
Positive?		YES	NO
Key Words			
Rephrase			
Rule Out Choices			
A	B	C	D

37

Angina

- Varies from mild to severe, transient to prolonged, gradual or sudden onset
- May radiate to either arm, shoulder, jaw, neck, or epigastric area
- Other S/S: dyspnea, tachycardia, palpitations, nausea and vomiting, fatigue, diaphoresis, pallor, syncope
- Usually subsides with rest or nitroglycerin
- Often precipitated by exercise, cold exposure, heavy meal, stress, intercourse

Diet Therapy

- Diet modification
- Goal is to reduce serum cholesterol and serum triglycerides
- Maintain ideal body weight
- Daily cholesterol intake should be restricted to <200 mg/day

Cholesterol-Lowering Drugs

- May be initiated if diet modification unsuccessful
  - Atorvastatin (Lipitor)
  - Lovastatin (Mevacor)
  - Pravastatin (Pravachol)
  - Rosuvastatin (Crestor)
  - Simvastatin (Zocor)
  - Ezetemibe (Zetia)
  - Gemfibrozil (Lopid)
  - Niacin (nicotinic acid)

Oxygen

- Administer at 4-6 L/min to assist in oxygenating myocardial tissue

Nitroglycerin

- Dilates the coronary arteries
- Increases blood flow to the damaged area of myocardium
- Dose:
  - 0.4 mg/tablet
  - 1 tab sublingual q 5 min × 3 doses

Morphine Sulfate

- Analgesic
- ↓ reduces Anxiety
- ↓ reduces Tachypnea
- Relaxes bronchial smooth muscle
- Improves gas exchange

Thrombolytic Therapy

- Useful when infarction is diagnosed early
- Streptokinase and tPA
  - Administered IV
  - Most effective if given within 6 hours of onset of chest pain
- Heparin therapy will usually follow thrombolytic therapy

Beta-Blockers

- Decrease heart rate
- Reduce workload of heart
- Decrease oxygen demand of myocardium

Reduction of Risk Factors

- Stop smoking
- Lose weight
- Decrease blood pressure
- Increase activity/exercise

Drug Therapy

- May be initiated if diet modification unsuccessful
- Antiplatelet
  - Acetylsalicylic acid (ASA)
  - Clopidogrel (Plavix)
- Beta-blockers
- Atenolol (Tenormin)
- Metoprolol (Lopressor, Toprol)
- Nitrates
  - Nitroglycerin
  - Nitroprusside
- Calcium channel blockers
  - Diltiazem (Cardizem)
  - Verapamil (Calan, Isoptin)
- Thrombolytics
  - Alteplase (recombinant t-PA) (Activase)
  - Reteplase (r-PA) (Retavase)
  - Tenecteplase (TNK-tPA)
  - Streptokinase (Streptase)
- Anticoagulants
  - Unfractionated heparin
  - Low-molecular-weight heparin (LMWH) (enoxaparin [Lovenox])
- Angiotensin-converting enzyme inhibitors
  - Captopril (Capoten)
  - Enalapril (Vasotec)
  - Benazepril (Lotensin)
- Analgesics
  - Morphine sulfate

Antiarrhythmic Medications

- Class I: sodium channel blockers (decrease conduction velocity in the atria, ventricles, and His-Purkinje system)
  IA
  - Disopyramide (Norpace)
  - Procainamide (Pronestyl)
  - Quinidine
  IB
  - Lidocaine (Xylocaine)
  - Mexiletine (Mexitil)
  - Phenytoin (Dilantin)
  - Tocainide (Tonocard)
  IC
  - Flecainide (Tambocor)
  - Propafenone (Rythmol)
- Other Class I
  - Moricizine (Ethmozine)
- Class II: β-adrenergic blockers (decrease automaticity of the SA node, decrease conduction velocity in AV node)
  - Acebutolol (Sectral)
  - Atenolol (Tenormin)
  - Esmolol (Brevibloc)
  - Metoprolol (Lopressor)
  - Sotalol (Betapace)

Calcium Channel Blockers

- Decrease conduction through AV node
- Slow heart rate
- Decrease oxygen demand by myocardium

Medical Interventions

- Percutaneous transluminal coronary angioplasty (PTCA)
  — Balloon angioplasty
- Intracoronary stents
- Coronary artery bypass graft (CABG)

Acute Myocardial Infarction

- Destruction of myocardial tissue due to lack of blood and oxygen supply
- Begins with an occlusion of coronary artery
- Ischemia, injury, infarction

Ischemia

- Results from reduced blood flow and oxygen to the coronary arteries
- If not reversed, then injury occurs
- Ischemia lasting 20 minutes or more is sufficient to produce irreversible tissue damage

Injury

Prolonged interruption of oxygen supply and nutrients
- Cells are still salvageable

Infarction

- Tissue necrosis and death
- Irreversible damage
- Scar tissue: has no electrical stimulation or contractility
- Within 24 hours of infarction the healing process begins

Complications

- Up to 90% of clients suffer complications, including
  — Dysrhythmias
  — Cardiac failure
  — Cardiogenic shock
  — Thromboembolism
  — Ventricular rupture

Signs and Symptoms

- Pain
  — Sudden-onset severity increases
  — May persist for hours or days not relieved by rest or nitroglycerine
  — Heavy/constrictive
  — Located behind the sternum
  — May radiate to arms, back, neck, or jaw
- Skin: cool and clammy
- Rapid, irregular, feeble pulse

Atypical Symptoms

- Women
  — Discomfort rather than pain
  — Shortness of breath
  — Extreme fatigue

- Class III: potassium channel blockers (delay repolarization)
  — Amiodarone (Cordarone)
  — Dofetilide (Tikosyn)
  — Sotalol (Betapace)
- Class IV: calcium channel blockers (decrease automaticity of SA node, delay AV node conduction)
  — Diltiazem (Cardizem)
  — Verapamil (Calan)
- Other antidysrhythmic drugs
  — Adenosine (Adenocard)
  — Digoxin (Lanoxin)
  — Ibutilide (Corvert)
  — Magnesium

- Diabetics
  - Asymptomatic
  - Neuropathy
  - Dyspnea
- Geriatrics
  - Confusion
  - Change in mental status
  - Dizziness
  - Shortness of breath

Medical Diagnosis
- ECG (12 lead)
- Confirm by lab tests
- Troponin
- Myoglobin
- Cardiac enzymes

Cardiac Lab Tests
- Troponin:
  - Found only in cardiac muscle
  - May present as early as 1 hour after injury
  - Peaks within 24 hours
  - Returns to normal in 5-14 days
- Myoglobin:
  - Released 1 hour after an acute myocardial infarction (MI)
  - Rises before creatine kinase-MB levels
  - Returns to normal within 24 hours
- Cardiac enzymes
  - With sustained ischemia, enzymes are released into the interstitial fluid
  - Are assessed at regular intervals to confirm acute MI

A client complains of a severe headache after receiving nitroglycerin 0.4 mg SL for angina. What prescription should the nurse administer?
A. A second dose of nitroglycerin
B. A scheduled dose of low-dose aspirin
C. A PRN dose of acetaminophen PO
D. A PRN dose of morphine sulfate IV

HESI Test Question Approach			
Positive?		YES	NO
Key Words			
Rephrase			
Rule Out Choices			
A	B	C	D

Treatment
- Overall goal is to preserve myocardial tissue
- Drug therapy
  - Oxygen
  - Nitroglycerine
  - Morphine
  - Thrombolytic therapy
  - Other medications
- Angioplasty and stents
  - Used when drug therapy is not successful
- Coronary artery bypass graft
  - Severe coronary artery disease detected
  - Can be emergent or elective

Dysrhythmias

- A standard ECG uses 12 leads.
  — Provides best overall evaluation
- Telemetry
  — Usually three leads show one view of the heart
- Holter monitor
  — Usually on for 24-hour continuous reading

Electrocardiogram (ECG)

- P wave
  — Atrial depolarization
- QRS complex
  — Ventricular depolarization
  — Normal <0.11 second
- ST segment
  — Early ventricular repolarization
- P–R interval
  — Time for impulse to travel through AV node
  — Normal 0.12 to 0.2 second
- R–R interval
  — Measure regularity of heartbeat

Dysrhythmias

- Client may be asymptomatic until cardiac output is altered
- May complain of palpitations, syncope, pain, dyspnea, diaphoresis
- Will display change in pulse rate/rhythm and ECG changes
- Always treat the client and *not* the monitor.

Atrial Dysrhythmias

- A-fib (atrial fibrillation)
  — Chaotic activity in the AV node
  — No true P waves visible
  — Irregular ventricular rhythm
  — Risk for CVA
- Anticoagulant therapy is needed
- Atrial flutter
  — Sawtoothed waveform
  — Fluttering in chest
  — Ventricular rhythm states regular
- May use cardioversion to treat either atrial dysrhythmia

Ventricular Dysrhythmias

- V-tach (ventricular tachycardia)
  — Wide bizarre QRS complex
  — Assess whether patient has a pulse
  — Is cardiac output impaired?
  — Prepare for synchronized cardioversion
  — Administer antiarrhythmic drugs
- V-fib (ventricular fibrillation)
  — Cardiac emergency
  — No cardiac output
  — Start cardiopulmonary resuscitation (CPR)
  — Defibrillate as quickly as possible
  — Administer antiarrhythmic drugs

Inflammatory Heart Disease

- Endocarditis
  - S/S: fever, murmur, heart failure symptoms
  - Infective endocarditis can lead to damaged heart valves
  - Administer antibiotics for 4-6 weeks
  - Teach about anticoagulant therapy
- Pericarditis
  - S/S: Pain—hurts more with deep breath, pericardial friction rub
  - Monitor for ST segment elevation
  - Monitor hemodynamic status

Valvular Heart Disease

- Valves may be unable to:
  - Fully open (stenosis)
  - Fully close (insufficiency or regurgitation)
- Causes
  - Rheumatic fever
  - Congenital heart disease
  - Syphilis
  - Endocarditis
  - Hypertension

Mitral Valve Stenosis

- Early period—may have no symptoms
- Later—excessive fatigue, dyspnea on exertion, orthopnea, dry cough, hemoptysis, or pulmonary edema
- Rumbling apical diastolic murmur and atrial fibrillation are common

Nursing Plans and Interventions

- See section on congestive heart failure
- Monitor of a-fib with thrombus formation
- Prophylactic antibiotic therapy before any invasive procedures (dental, surgical, childbirth)
- May require surgical repair or valve replacement
- Teaching concerning need for lifelong anticoagulant therapy if valve replacement done

The nurse receives report on four clients on the cardiac unit. Which client should the nurse assess first? The client who has

A. Thrombophlebitis and a positive Homans sign
B. Left-sided heart failure and an S3 gallop
C. Pericarditis and inspiratory chest pain
D. Halo vision after digitalization

HESI Test Question Approach			
Positive?		YES	NO
Key Words			
Rephrase			
Rule Out Choices			
A	B	C	D

Vascular Disorders

Arterial

- Smooth shiny skin
- Pallor on elevation
- Weak peripheral pulses
- Sharp or tingling pain
- Cool to touch
- Intermittent claudication (classic symptom)
- Painful, nonedematous ulcers

Venous

- Monitor for history of deep vein thrombosis
- Bluish purple skin discoloration
- Normal peripheral pulses
- Warm to touch
- Slightly painful ulcers with marked edema

Nursing Interventions and Treatment

General

- Change positions frequently; avoid sitting with crossed legs
- Wear *no* restrictive clothing
- Keep extremities warm with clothing, not external heaters
- Discourage smoking
- Thrombolytic agents if thrombosis

Abdominal Aortic Aneurysm

- Pulsating abdominal mass
- Bruit heard over abdomen
- Confirmed on radiograph
- If ruptures: S/S of hypovolemic shock
- Surgical repair of aneurysm postoperative care
  - Monitor for S/S of renal failure, postoperative ileus
  - Changes in pulses, S/S of occluded graft

Thrombophlebitis

- Inflammation of the venous wall with clot formation
- S/S: calf pain, + Homans sign, edema of calf
- Restrict ambulation
- Elevate extremity
- Antiembolic stockings
- Medications
  - Heparin therapy
    - Monitor partial thromboplastin time (PTT)
  - Coumadin therapy
    - Monitor prothrombin time (PT), international normalized ratio (INR)
  - Antiplatelet agents
    - Ticlid
    - Plavix

Arterial

- Bed rest
- Topical antibiotics
- Surgical intervention

Venous

- Systemic antibiotics
- Compression dressing
- Limb elevation

Which client should the nurse assess first? A client receiving

A. Oxygen per nasal cannula who is dyspneic with mild exertion and has a hemoglobin of 7 g/dL
B. IV aminoglycosides per CVC who complains of nausea and has a trough level below therapeutic levels
C. Packed RBCs who complains of flank pain and has a BP of 98/52 mm Hg
D. Chemotherapy whose temperature is 98.9° F and has a WBC count of 2500/mm^3

HESI Test Question Approach			
Positive?		YES	NO
Key Words			
Rephrase			
Rule Out Choices			
A	B	C	D

Nursing Plans and Interventions

- Treatment of underlying pathology
- Administer blood products as ordered
- Diet should be high in iron-rich foods, folic acid, vitamin B_{12}, vitamin B_6, amino acids, and vitamin C
- Parenteral iron is given using Z-track technique

5 Ingestion, Digestion, Absorption, and Elimination

The nurse is ordering afternoon snacks for several clients. Which client will benefit from a milk shake with whole milk and added protein powder? The client who has
A. Cirrhosis
B. Paralytic ileus
C. Cholelithiasis
D. Dumping syndrome

HESI Test Question Approach		
Positive?	YES	NO
Key Words		
Rephrase		
Rule Out Choices		
A	B	C	D

Gastroesophageal Reflux Disease (GERD)

- Not a disease but a syndrome
- Any clinically significant symptomatic condition secondary to reflux of gastric contents into the lower esophagus
- Most common upper GI problem seen in adults

Etiology and Pathophysiology

There is no one single cause of GERD.
- Predisposing conditions
  — Hiatal hernia
  — Incompetent lower esophageal sphincter (LES)
  — Decreased esophageal clearance (ability to clear liquids or food from the esophagus into the stomach) resulting from impaired esophageal motility
  — Decreased gastric emptying

Nursing Assessment

- Heartburn after eating
- Fullness and discomfort after eating
- Ask client what foods seem to aggravate symptoms
- Positive diagnosis from barium swallow or fluoroscopy (hiatal hernia)

Nursing Plans and Interventions

- Encourage small frequent meals
- Sit up while eating and remain upright for 1 hour after eating
- Stop eating 3 hours before bedtime
- Elevate head of bed 4-6 inches

Peptic Ulcer Disease

- Significant gastric ulcers are caused by *Helicobacter pylori* bacteria.

45

- Risk factors include:
  — Drugs: NSAIDs, corticosteroids
  — Alcohol
  — Cigarette smoking
  — Trauma

Nursing Assessment
- Left epigastric pain, may radiate to back
- Epigastric pain relieved with food
- Diagnosed with
  — Barium swallow
  — Upper endoscopy

Nursing Plans and Interventions
- Onset of symptoms?
- What relieves symptoms?
- Monitor stools for color, consistency, occult blood
- Administer antacids and antibiotics as ordered
- Avoid caffeine
- Small frequent meals are best

Complications
- Uncontrolled bleeding
  — Prepare for immediate surgery
- Dumping syndrome postoperative complication
  — Occurs 5 to 30 minutes after eating
  — Vertigo, syncope, tachycardia
  — Small frequent meals
  — High-fat, high-protein, low-CHO diet
  — Avoid liquids with meals

Client Teaching
- Avoid medications such as:
  — Salicylates
  — NSAIDs
- Inform healthcare personnel of history of peptic ulcer disease
- Symptoms of GI bleeding:
  — Dark tarry stools
  — Coffee ground emesis
  — Bright red rectal bleeding

Lower GI Problems
Crohn's Disease
- Affects both small and large intestine
- Right lower quadrant abdominal pain
- Nausea and vomiting
- Diarrhea, fatty stools
- Barium enema shows narrowing with areas of strictures separated by segments of normal bowels

Interventions
- Initial treatment is based on symptomatic relief, which usually includes parenteral replacement of fluids, electrolytes, and blood products. Complete bed rest and assistance with ADL during acute phases are prescribed.

- Pharmacotherapy
  — Sedatives and tranquilizers: To promote rest and reduce anxiety
  — Antidiarrheal medications: To decrease diarrhea and cramping
  — Sulfasalazine: To treat acute exacerbations of colonic and ileocolonic disease
  — Corticosteroids: To reduce the active inflammatory response
  — Immunosuppressive agents: To allow dosage reduction or withdrawal of corticosteroids
  — Antibiotics: To control infections and perianal fistulas
- Nutritional management
  — During acute exacerbations, TPN and NPO
  — Elemental diet
  — Bland diets
  — No milk, milk products
  — Supplementation of vitamins and minerals, especially calcium, iron, folate, magnesium, vitamin D
- Surgical management is reserved for complications rather than used as a primary form of therapy. Common indications for surgery include bowel obstruction, internal and enterocutaneous fistulas, intraabdominal abscesses, and perianal disease.

Ulcerative Colitis
- Occurs in large bowel and rectum
- Symptoms
  — Diarrhea
  — Abdominal pain
  — Liquid stools, 10 to 20/day
  — Anemia
- Interventions
  — Low-residue, low-fat, high-protein, high-calorie diet
  — No dairy products
  — Tepid fluids
  — Daily calorie count
  — Monitor I & O

Diverticular Diseases
- Left lower quadrant pain
- S/S of intestinal obstruction
  — Abdominal distention
  — Constipation/diarrhea
- + Barium enema
- Colonoscopy

Nursing Interventions
- High-fiber diet unless inflammation is present
- If inflammation present
  — NPO
  — Then low residue, bland diet
  — Bulk-forming laxatives
  — Avoid heavy lifting, tight clothing, and straining

Intestinal Obstruction

- Mechanical causes
  - Adhesions most common
  - Strangulated hernia
  - Tumors
- Neurogenic causes
  - Paralytic ileus
  - Spinal cord lesion
- Vascular cause
  - Mesenteric artery occlusion

Nursing Assessment

- Sudden abdominal pain
- History of obstruction
- High-pitched bowel sounds with early mechanical obstruction
- Bowel sounds diminished or absent with neurogenic or late mechanical obstruction

Nursing Interventions

- NPO
- IV fluids
- Nasogastric tube to intermittent suction

LIVER, PANCREAS, AND BILIARY TRACT PROBLEMS

Cirrhosis

- Degeneration of the liver tissue
- A chronic progressive disease

Nursing Assessment

- Early sign: RUQ pain
- History of
  - ETOH abuse
  - Street drug abuse
- Jaundice
- Fruity or musty breath
- Asterixis
- Palmar erythema
- Ascites
- Weight loss

Esophageal Varices

- Esophageal varices may rupture.

Treatment

- Esophagogastric balloon
- Blakemore-Sengstaken tube
- Vitamin K
- Blood products
- Coagulation factors

Nursing Interventions

- Monitor for bleeding
  - Avoid injections
  - Maintain pressure for 5 minutes after venipunctures

- Provide skin care
  — Avoid soap
  — Apply lotions
- Monitor fluid and electrolytes
  — Accurate I & O
  — Weigh daily
  — Restrict fluids (1500 mL/day)
  — Abdominal girth

Dietary Teaching
- Protein may need to be restricted
- Low sodium
- Low potassium
- Low fat
- High carbohydrate
- May need to take lactulose (Cephulac) as ammonia detoxicant/stimulant laxative

Hepatitis
Nursing Assessment
- Fatigue, weakness
- Anorexia, nausea
- Jaundice
- Dark urine
- Joint pain, muscle aches

Pancreatitis
- Acute: autodigestion of the pancreas
  — Alcohol ingestion and biliary tract disease are major causes.
- Chronic: progressive, destructive disease
  — Long-term alcohol use is major factor in disease.

Acute Pancreatitis Assessment
Abdominal pain is the predominant symptom of acute pancreatitis
- Located in the left upper quadrant
- Radiates to the back
- Sudden onset
- Described as severe, deep, piercing, and continuous
- Aggravated by eating and is not relieved by vomiting
- Accompanied by flushing, cyanosis, and dyspnea

Other Manifestations of Acute Pancreatitis
- Nausea and vomiting
- Low-grade fever
- Leukocytosis
- Jaundice
- Abdominal tenderness with muscle guarding
- Bowel sounds may be decreased or absent and ileus may occur
- Areas of ecchymoses *Grey Turner spots* or *sign,* a bluish flank discoloration and *Cullen sign,* a bluish periumbilical discoloration
- Hypotension
- Tachycardia
- Hypovolemia (massive fluid shift into the retroperitoneal space)

- Shock (hemorrhage into the pancreas)
- Toxemia (activated pancreatic enzymes)
- The lungs are frequently involved (crackles)

Chronic Pancreatitis Assessment

- Steatorrhea
- Diarrhea
- Jaundice
- Ascites
- Weight loss

Nursing Plans and Interventions

- Acute management
  - NPO
  - NG tube to suction
  - Morphine for pain management
  - Sitting up or leaning forward may reduce pain
  - Monitor blood sugar
  - Teach foods and fluids to avoid
- Chronic management
  - Pain management
    - Morphine
  - Pancreatic enzymes
    - Creon
    - Viokase
    - Mix powdered forms with fruit juice or apple-sauce; avoid mixing with proteins
  - Teach foods and fluids to avoid

A client who has an obstruction of the common bile duct caused by cholelithiasis passes clay-colored stools containing streaks of fat. What action should the nurse implement?
A. Auscultate for diminished bowel sounds
B. Send a stool specimen to the lab
C. Document the assessment in the chart
D. Notify the healthcare provider

HESI Test Question Approach		
Positive?	YES	NO
Key Words		
Rephrase		
Rule Out Choices		
A	B	C	D

Cholecystitis and Cholelithiasis

- Cholecystitis: acute inflammation of the gallbladder
- Cholelithiasis: formation or presence of gallstones

Nursing Assessment

- Pain
- Fever
- Elevated WBCs
- Abdominal tenderness
- Jaundice

Nursing Plans and Interventions

- Analgesics for pain
- NPO
- NG to suction

50

- IV antibiotics
- Low-fat diet
  — Avoid fried, spicy, and fatty foods

Treatment
- Cholecystitis
  — IV hydration
  — Administer antibiotics
  — Pain management
- Cholelithiasis
  — Nonsurgical removal
    • Endoscopic retrograde cholangiopancreatography (ERCP)
    • Lithotripsy
  — Surgical approach
    • Cholecystectomy, laparoscopic or open

A client is admitted with gastric ulcer disease and GI bleeding. Which risk factor should the nurse identify in the client's history?
A. Eats heavily seasoned foods
B. Uses NSAIDs daily
C. Consumes alcohol every day
D. Follows an acid-ash diet

HESI Test Question Approach		
Positive?	YES	NO
Key Words		
Rephrase		
Rule Out Choices		
A	B	C	D

RENAL AND UROLOGIC PROBLEMS

Urinary Tract Infections
- Obtain clean-catch midstream specimen
- Administer antibiotics as ordered
  — Take fully prescribed dose
  — Do not skip doses
- Encourage fluid intake of 3000 mL/day
- Encourage voiding every 2 to 3 hours

Urinary Tract Obstruction
- Caused by calculi or stones
- Location of pain can help locate stone
  — Flank pain (stone usually in upper ureter)
  — Pain radiating to abdomen (stone likely in ureter or bladder)
- Nursing plan
  — Administer narcotics
  — Strain all urine
  — Encourage high fluid intake
    • 3 to 4 L/day
  — Strict I & O
  — May need surgical management

Benign Prostatic Hyperplasia

- Enlargement of the prostate
  - Most common treatment: transurethral resection of the prostate (TURP)
  - Can be done with laser to burn out prostate
  - If prostate is too large, will use suprapubic approach
  - Assess for
    - Increased urinary frequency/decreased output
    - Bladder distention (increases risk of spasm)

Nursing Plans and Interventions

- Preoperative teaching
  - Pain management
  - Oversized balloon catheter
- Bladder spasms
  - Common after surgery
  - Use antispasmodics
    - Belladonna and opium suppositories
    - Ditropan
    - Bentyl
- Continuous bladder irrigation is typically done to remove blood clots and ensure drainage
- Drainage should be reddish pink for 24 hours, clearing to light pink
- Monitor color and amount of urine output
- Notify physician if client has bright red bleeding with large clots

Discharge Teaching

- Continue to drink 12 to 14 glasses of water per day
- Avoid straining
- Avoid strenuous activity, sports, lifting, and intercourse for 3 to 4 weeks
- Report large amounts of blood or frank blood

The charge nurse is making assignments on the renal unit. Which client should the nurse assign to an LPN who is new to the unit?

A. An older client who is draining thick, dark, red drainage in a urinary catheter 1 day after a transurethral prostatic resection

B. A middle-aged client admitted with acute renal failure secondary to reaction to IVP dye

C. An older client who has end-stage renal disease and complains of nausea after receiving Lanoxin

D. A middle-aged client who receives hemodialysis and is prescribed epoetin alfa (Epogen) subcutaneous daily

HESI Test Question Approach			
Positive?		YES	NO
Key Words			
Rephrase			
Rule Out Choices			
A	B	C	D

A client who has acute renal failure is admitted and the potassium level is 6.4 mEq/L. Which snack should the nurse offer?

A. An orange
B. A milk shake
C. Dried fruit and nuts
D. A gelatin dessert

<table>
<tr><td colspan="5">HESI Test Question Approach</td></tr>
<tr><td>Positive?</td><td></td><td></td><td>YES</td><td>NO</td></tr>
<tr><td>Key Words</td><td></td><td></td><td></td><td></td></tr>
<tr><td></td><td></td><td></td><td></td><td></td></tr>
<tr><td></td><td></td><td></td><td></td><td></td></tr>
<tr><td>Rephrase</td><td></td><td></td><td></td><td></td></tr>
<tr><td></td><td></td><td></td><td></td><td></td></tr>
<tr><td></td><td></td><td></td><td></td><td></td></tr>
<tr><td colspan="5">Rule Out Choices</td></tr>
<tr><td>A</td><td>B</td><td>C</td><td>D</td><td></td></tr>
</table>

Acute Renal Failure (ARF)

- A reversible syndrome if symptoms are caught early enough
- Remember:
  - Kidneys use 25% of normal cardiac output to maintain function.
  - Kidneys excrete 1 to 2 L of urine per 24 hours for adults.
  - Three types of ARF
    - Prerenal
    - Intrarenal
    - Postrenal

Prerenal Failure

- Etiological factors
  - Hemorrhage
  - Hypovolemia
  - Decreased cardiac output
  - Decreased renal perfusion

Intrarenal Failure

- Etiological factors
  - May develop secondary to prerenal failure
  - Nephrotoxins
  - Infections (glomerulonephritis)
  - Renal injury
  - Vascular lesions

Postrenal Failure

- Etiological factors for obstruction
  - Calculi
  - Benign prostatic hyperplasia (BPH)
  - Tumors
  - Strictures

Nursing Assessment

- Decreased urine output
- Weight gain
- Edema
- Diagnostic test results: oliguric phase
  - ↓ Urine output
  - ↑ BUN (blood urea nitrogen) and creatinine
  - ↑ Potassium

53

- — ↓ Sodium (serum)
- — ↓ pH
- — Metabolic acidosis
- — ↑ Urine sodium
- — Fixed at 1.010, specific gravity
- Diagnostic test results: diuretic phase
  - — ↑ Urine output
  - — ↓ Fluid volume
  - — ↓ Potassium
  - — ↓ Sodium
  - — ↓ Urine specific gravity
  - — ↓ Urine sodium

Nursing Plans and Interventions

- In oliguric phase give only enough fluids to replace losses + 400 to 500 mL/24 hr
- Strict I & O
- Monitor lab values closely
- Watch for ECG changes
- Monitor weight daily

After hemodialysis, the nurse is evaluating the blood results for a client who has end-stage renal disease. Which value should the nurse verify with the laboratory?
A. Elevated serum potassium
B. Increase in serum calcium
C. Low hemoglobin
D. Reduction in serum sodium

HESI Test Question Approach		
Positive?	YES	NO
Key Words		
Rephrase		
Rule Out Choices		
A	B	C	D

Chronic Kidney Disease (CKD)

- End-stage renal disease
- Progressive irreversible damage to the nephrons and glomeruli
- Causes
  - — Diabetic nephropathy
  - — Hypertensive nephrosclerosis
  - — Glomerulonephritis
  - — Polycystic kidney disease

Nursing Assessment

- Early stage
  - — Polyuria
  - — Renal insufficiency
- Late stage
  - — Oliguria
  - — Hematuria
  - — Proteinuria
  - — Edema

— Increased BP
— Muscle wasting, secondary to negative nitrogen balance
— Ammonia taste in mouth
— ↑ Creatinine, ↑ phosphorus, ↑ potassium
■ End stage
— Anuria (<100 mL/24 hr)

Nursing Plans and Interventions
■ Monitor serum electrolytes
■ Weigh daily
■ Strict I & O
■ Renal diet
— Low protein
— Low sodium
— Low potassium
— Low phosphate

Medications
■ Drugs to manage the associated complications
— Aluminum hydroxide (to bind phosphates)
— Epoetin (Epogen) (to treat anemia)
— Antihypertensive therapy
— Calcium supplements and vitamin D
— Antihyperlipidemics
— Statins (to lower LDL)
— Fibrates (to lower triglycerides)
■ CAUTION: As kidney function decreases, medication doses need adjustment.

Renal Dialysis
■ Hemodialysis
— AV fistula
■ Ø Venipunctures, Ø IVs, Ø BP in AV shunt arm
■ Withhold medications that would affect hemodynamic stability before dialysis
■ Peritoneal dialysis
— Monitor indwell and outflow times closely
— Monitor I & O

Postoperative Care: Kidney Surgery
■ Respiratory status
— Auscultate to detect "wet" sounds
— Demonstrate splinting method
■ Circulatory status
— Monitor for shock
— Monitor surgical site for bleeding
■ Pain relief status
— Administer narcotic analgesics as needed
■ Urinary status
— Check urinary output and drainage from *all* tubes
— Strict I & O

55

A client with a 20-year history of type 1 diabetes mellitus is having renal function tests because of recent fatigue, weakness, a blood urea nitrogen (BUN) of 24 mg/dL, and serum creatinine of 1.6 mg/dL. What further inquiry should the nurse make related to early symptoms of renal insufficiency?

A. Dyspnea
B. Nocturia
C. Confusion
D. Stomatitis

HESI Test Question Approach		
Positive?	YES	NO
Key Words		
Rephrase		
Rule Out Choices		
A	B	C	D

6 Regulatory, Reproductive, and Urinary Systems

A male client who has type 1 diabetes returns to the clinic for follow-up after dietary counseling. The client states that he has been managing his diabetes very closely. Which lab result indicates the client is maintaining tight control of the disease?
A. FBS changes from 135 to 110 mg/dL.
B. SMBG at HS changes from 45 to 90.
C. Glycosylated Hgb changes from 9% to 6%.
D. Urine ketones change from 0 to 3.

HESI Test Question Approach			
Positive?		YES	NO
Key Words			
Rephrase			
Rule Out Choices			
A	B	C	D

Metabolic Syndrome/Obesity

- Assessment
- Interventions
  — Gastric bypass
  — Lap band

Prediabetes is a condition where individuals are at an increased risk for developing diabetes. In this condition, the blood glucose levels are high but not high enough to meet the diagnostic criteria for diabetes.

Diabetes mellitus is a chronic multisystem disease related to abnormal insulin production, impaired insulin use, or both.

- Type 1 diabetes: immune-mediated disease. The body's own T cells destroy pancreatic beta cells, which are the source of insulin.
- In type 2 diabetes: the pancreas continues to produce some insulin but, it is either insufficient for the needs of the body or is poorly used by the tissues, or both.

Clinical Manifestations

- Type 1
  — The onset of type 1 diabetes is rapid
  — The initial manifestations are usually acute
  — The classic symptoms are polyuria, polydipsia, and polyphagia.
  — Weight loss may occur as the body cannot get glucose.
  — Weakness and fatigue may also be experienced
  — Ketoacidosis may occur
- Type 2
  — The clinical manifestations of type 2 diabetes are often nonspecific.
  — More common manifestations include:
  — Fatigue

57

— Recurrent infections
  • Vaginal yeast
  • Candidal infections
— Prolonged wound healing
— Visual changes

Because type 2 diabetes is asymptomatic in the early phases, it is recommended that high-risk people be screened annually for diabetes.

Diabetes Mellitus
Nursing Assessment

■ Integument: skin breakdown
■ Eyes: retinal problems, cataracts
■ Kidneys: edema, urinary retention
■ Periphery: cool skin
■ Ulcerations on extremities and thick nails
■ Cardiopulmonary angina and dyspnea

Nursing Plans and Interventions

■ Teach injection techniques
■ Refrigerate unopened insulin
■ Diet
  — 55%-60% carbohydrate
  — 12%-15% protein
  — 30% fat
■ Exercise regimen
■ Plan meals and snacks around exercise routine
■ May need snack before or during exercise
■ Monitor for S/S of hypoglycemia
■ Foot care
  — Check daily
  — Report signs of injury
■ Manage sick days
  — Keep taking insulin
  — Check blood sugar more frequently
  — Watch for S/S of hyperglycemia

Oral Agents

Oral agents are not insulin; they work on the three defects of type 2 diabetes:
1. Insulin resistance
2. Decreased insulin production
3. Increased hepatic glucose production

Sulfonylureas: increase insulin production from the pancreas, therefore hypoglycemia is the major side effect with sulfonylureas.
■ glipizide (Glucotrol, Glucotrol XL)
■ glyburide (Micronase, DiaBeta, Glynase)
■ glimepiride (Amaryl)

Meglitinides: increase insulin production from the pancreas. They are more rapidly absorbed and eliminated than sulfonylureas, therefore are less likely to cause hypoglycemia.
■ repaglinide (Prandin)
■ nateglinide (Starlix)

Biguanides: reduce glucose production by the liver. They also enhance insulin sensitivity at the tissue level. The first-choice drug for most people with type 2 diabetes. Do not use in patients with kidney disease, liver disease, heart failure, or people who drink excessive amounts of alcohol.

α-Glucosidase inhibitors: (starch blockers) Slow down the absorption of carbohydrate in the small intestine.
- acarbose (Precose)
- miglitol (Glyset)

Thiazolidinediones: (insulin sensitizers) most effective for people who have insulin resistance. Will not cause hypoglycemia when used alone
- pioglitazone (Actos)
- rosiglitazone (Avandia); Do not use in patients with heart failure. Increased risk of myocardial infarction and stroke.

Dipeptidyl Peptidase-4 (DPP-4) inhibitor: inhibits DPP-4, thus slowing the inactivation of incretin hormones. Since the DPP-4 inhibitors are glucose dependent, they lower the potential for hypoglycemia.
- sitagliptin (Januvia)
- saxagliptin (Onglyza)

Incretin mimetic: simulate one of the incretin hormones found to be decreased in people with type 2 diabetes. It is administered using a subcutaneous injection in a prefilled pen. Acute pancreatitis and kidney problems have been associated with its use.
- Exenatide (Byetta)
- liraglutide (Victoza)

Amylin analog: It is a synthetic analog of human amylin. It is indicated for type 1 diabetics and type 2 diabetics who have not achieved glucose control despite taking insulin at mealtimes. It is administered subcutaneously and cannot be mixed with insulin. It can cause severe hypoglycemia when used with insulin.
- Pramlintide (Symlin)

Insulin Pharmacokinetics after SC Injection
Rapid acting insulin:
1. glulisine (Apidra). Given within 15 minutes of meal.
   a. Onset: 0.25 hr
   b. Peak: 1 hr
   c. Duration: 2-3 hr
2. lispro (Humalog). Given within 15 minutes of meal.
   a. Onset: 0.25 hr
   b. Peak: 1 hr
   c. Duration: 4 hr
3. aspart (NovoLog). Given within 15 minutes of meal.
   a. Onset: 0.50 hr
   b. Peak: 1-3 hr
   c. Duration: 3-5 hr
4. regular (Humulin R). Given within 30 minutes of meal.
   a. Onset: 0.50 - 1 hr
   b. Peak: 2-4 hr
   c. Duration: 5-7 hr

HESI Hint

Insulin dose reductions may be needed if the client has kidney or liver impairment since insulin is excreted by the kidneys and is metabolized by the liver.

Intermediate acting insulin: Not to be given IV. Can be mixed with rapid-acting insulins. (See combinations below)
1. Neutral Protamine Hagedorn - NPH (Humulin H)
    a. Onset: 3-4 hr
    b. Peak: 6-12 hr
    c. Duration: 18-28 hr

Long-acting insulin: Cannot be mixed with any other type of insulin. Usually given once a day in the morning. Acts as basal insulin. Do not shake solutions. CAUTION: Solution is clear; do not confuse with regular insulin.
1. glargine (Lantus)
    a. Onset: 1-5 hr
    b. Peak: Plateau
    c. Duration: 24 hr
2. detemir (Levemir)
    a. Onset: 3-4 hr
    b. Peak: Peakless
    c. Duration: 24 hr

Combinations (Premix Insulins)
1. NPH and regular: 70/30 (70% NPH insulin and 30% regular insulin)
    a. Onset: 0.5-1 hr
    b. Peak: 1.5-12 hr
    c. Duration: Up to 24 hr
2. Lispro insulins: 75/25 (75% insulin lispro protamine suspension and 25% insulin lispro)
    a. Onset: 0.25-0.5 hr
    b. Peak: ≥ 2 hr
    c. Duration: Approx. 22 hr
3. Lispro insulins: 50/50 (50% insulin lispro protamine suspension and 50% insulin lispro)
    a. Onset: 0.25-0.5 hr
    b. Peak: 0.5-1.5 hr
    c. Duration: Approx. 22 hr
4. Aspart insulins: 70/30 (70% insulin aspart protamine suspension and 30% insulin aspart)
    a. Onset: .17-.33 hr
    b. Peak: 1-4 hr
    c. Duration: Up to 24 hr

Given the rapid onset of the analog premixed insulin, it should be given shortly before meals, and not at bedtime. Patients who choose to use the premixed insulin preparations should have fairly routine lifestyles.

OTHER ENDOCRINE PROBLEMS

Which client should the nurse assess first? A client who has

A. Hyperthyroidism exhibiting exophthalmos

B. Diabetes type 1 with an inflamed foot ulcer

C. Cushing's syndrome exhibiting moon faces

D. Addison's disease with tremors and diaphoresis

Thyroid Gland Feedback Loop

Hypothalamus

⇩

TRH (+)

Anterior Pituitary

T_3 & T_4 (−) TSH (+)

Thyroid Gland

Hyperthyroidism

Nursing Assessment

- Enlarged thyroid gland
- Exophthalmos
- Weight loss
- T_3 elevated
- T_4 elevated
- Diarrhea
- Tachycardia
- Bruit over thyroid

Nursing Plans and Interventions

Diet: high protein, high calorie, low caffeine, low fiber

- Treatment may trigger hypothyroidism, may need hormone replacement
- Propylthiouracil (PTU) therapy to block the synthesis of T_3 and T_4
- Iodine (131I) therapy to destroy thyroid cells

Surgical Management

- Thyroidectomy
- Check behind neck for drainage
- Support neck when moving client
- Assess for laryngeal edema
- Have tracheotomy set, oxygen, and suction equipment at bedside
- Have calcium gluconate at bedside

Which adaptation of the environment is most important for the nurse to include in the plan of care for a client with myxedema?

A. Reduce environmental stimuli

B. Prevent direct sunlight entering the room

C. Maintain a warm room temperature

D. Minimize exposure to visitors

HESI Test Question Approach			
Positive?		YES	NO
Key Words			
Rephrase			
Rule Out Choices			
A	B	C	D

HESI Test Question Approach			
Positive?		YES	NO
Key Words			
Rephrase			
Rule Out Choices			
A	B	C	D

Hypothyroidism

- Fatigue
- Bradycardia
- Weight gain
- Constipation
- Periorbital edema
- Cold intolerance
- Low T_3 (<70)
- Low T_4 (<5)

Nursing Plans and Interventions

Myxedema coma: an acute exacerbation of hypothyroidism; maintain airway

Teach medication regimen

Monitor for side effects of medications

Monitor bowel program for S/S of constipation

Thyroid Preparations

- Levothyroxine (Synthroid)
  — Monitor heart rate
  — Hold for pulse >100 beats/min
- Liothyronine (Cytomel)
  — Increase metabolic rate
  — Act as synthetic T_4
  — Check hormone levels regularly
  — Avoid food containing iodine
- Levothyroxine (T_4) + liothyronine (T_3) (Liotrix)
  — Fast onset

A client who is diagnosed with Addison's crisis is admitted, and the nurse places a peripheral saline lock. Which prescription should the nurse administer?

A. Calcium
B. Glucose
C. Potassium
D. Iodine

HESI Test Question Approach			
Positive?		YES	NO
Key Words			
Rephrase			
Rule Out Choices			
A	B	C	D

Addison's Disease

- Etiology
  — Sudden withdrawal from corticosteroids
  — Hypofunction of adrenal cortex
  — Lack of pituitary ACTH
- Signs and symptoms
  — Weight loss
  — N/V
  — Hypovolemia
  — Hypoglycemia
  — Hyponatremia
  — Hyperkalemia
  — Loss of body hair
  — Postural hypotension
  — Hyperpigmentation

Nursing Plans and Interventions

- Frequent vital signs
- Weigh daily
- Monitor serum electrolytes
- Diet: high sodium, low potassium, high carbohydrates
- Encourage at least 3 L of fluid per day

Cushing's Syndrome

Excess adrenal corticoid activity caused by adrenal, pituitary, or hypothalamus tumors

Nursing Assessment

- Moon face and edema of lower extremities
- Flat affect
- Obesity
- Abdominal striae
- Buffalo hump (fat deposits)
- Muscle atrophy, weakness
- Thin dry pale skin
- Hypertension
- Osteoporosis
- Immunosuppressed
- Hypervolemic
- Hirsutism
- Lab results
  — Hyperglycemia
  — Hypercalcemia
  — Hypernatremia
  — Hypokalemia
  — Increased plasma cortisol levels

Nursing Plans and Interventions

- Monitor for S/S of infection
- Fever
- Skin lesions
- Elevated WBCs
- Diet:
  — Low sodium
  — Low carbohydrate

Sexually Transmitted Diseases (STDs)

- Symptoms and treatment
  — Vary by disease
- Teach safer sex
  — Limit number of partners
  — Use latex condoms
- Report incidence of STDs to appropriate health agencies

Refer to Review Manuals for more in-depth information about STDs:

- *HESI Comprehensive Review for the NCLEX-RN Examination*
- *Mosby's Comprehensive Review of Nursing for NCLEX-RN Examination*
- *Saunders Comprehensive Review for the NCLEX-RN Examination*

FEMALE REPRODUCTIVE PROBLEMS

A 52-year-old who had an abdominal hysterectomy for a grade III severe dysplasia Pap smear is preparing for discharge. Which recommendation should the nurse offer the client about women's health and screening examinations?

A. Continue your annual Pap smears, mammogram, clinical breast examinations, and continue monthly breast self-examinations (BSE).

B. A Pap smear is no longer necessary, but continue annual mammogram and clinical breast examinations, plus monthly BSE.

C. Without ovaries, only an annual mammogram and clinical breast examinations are necessary.

D. Annual mammograms are not needed if biannual clinical breast examinations and weekly BSE are done.

Benign Uterine Tumors

- Arise from muscle tissue of the uterus
- Signs and symptoms:
  — Menorrhagia
  — Uterine enlargement
  — Dysmenorrhea
  — Anemia secondary to menorrhagia
  — Uterine enlargement
  — Low back pain and pelvic pain
  — Tend to disappear after menopause
- Surgical options:
  — Myomectomy
  — Hysterectomy
- Fertility issues

After stopping hormone replacement therapy (HRT), a 76-year-old reports she is experiencing increased vaginal discomfort during intercourse. What action should the nurse implement?

A. Suggest the use of a vaginal cream or lubricant
B. Recommend abstaining from sexual intercourse
C. Teach Kegel exercises daily
D. Instruct her to resume HRT

Uterine Prolapse, Cystocele, and Rectocele

- Preventive measures
  — Postpartum perineal exercises (Kegel)
  — Spaced pregnancy
  — Weight control
- Differing S/S for each condition
- Surgical intervention
  — Hysterectomy
  — Anterior and posterior vaginal repair
- Pain management postoperative
- Monitor urinary output postoperative
- Observe for S/S of bleeding and infection postoperative

HESI Test Question Approach		
Positive?	YES	NO
Key Words		
Rephrase		
Rule Out Choices		
A	B	C	D

HESI Test Question Approach		
Positive?	YES	NO
Key Words		
Rephrase		
Rule Out Choices		
A	B	C	D

A client who had a vaginal hysterectomy the previous day is saturating perineal pads with blood and requires frequent changes during the night. What priority action should the nurse implement?
A. Provide iron-rich foods on each dietary tray
B. Monitor the client's vital signs every hour
C. Administer IV fluids at the prescribed rate
D. Encourage postoperative leg exercises

HESI Test Question Approach			
Positive?		YES	NO
Key Words			
Rephrase			
Rule Out Choices			
A	B	C	D

MALE REPRODUCTIVE PROBLEMS

Etiology and Pathophysiology

Prostatitis is one of the most common urologic disorders. The four categories of prostatitis syndromes are:
- Acute bacterial prostatitis
- Chronic bacterial prostatitis
- Chronic prostatitis/chronic pelvic pain syndrome
- Asymptomatic inflammatory prostatitis

Common manifestations of acute bacterial prostatitis include:
- Fever
- Chills
- Back pain
- Perineal pain
- Dysuria
- Urinary frequency
- Urgency
- Cloudy urine

Diagnostic Studies
- Urinalysis (UA)
- Urine culture
- White blood cells (WBCs)
- Blood cultures
- PSA test (may be done to rule out prostate cancer)

Management
- Antibiotics
  - trimethoprim and sulfamethoxazole (Bactrim)
  - ciprofloxacin (Cipro)
  - ofloxacin (Floxin)
  - doxycycline (Vibramycin)
  - tetracycline
- Antiinflammatory agents for pain control
- Nursing interventions: encourage fluid intake

Problems of the Penis

- Hypospadias: the urethral meatus is located on the ventral surface of the penis.
- Epispadias: an opening of the urethra on the dorsal surface of the penis
  — Associated with other genitourinary tract defects
  — Surgery is usually done in early childhood.

Problems of Erectile Mechanism

Priapism: a painful erection lasting longer than 6 hours. Caused by an obstruction of the venous outflow in the penis. The condition may constitute a medical emergency.

Causes

- Thrombosis of the corpora cavernosal veins
- Leukemia
- Sickle cell anemia
- Diabetes mellitus
- Degenerative lesions of the spine
- Neoplasms of the brain or spinal cord

Treatment

- Sedatives
- Injection of smooth muscle relaxants directly into the penis
- Aspiration and irrigation of the corpora cavernosa with a large-bore needle
- Shunt to drain the corpora
  Complications include penile tissue necrosis.

Problems of the Scrotum and Testes

- Epididymitis: an acute, painful inflammatory process of the epididymis, due to an infectious process, trauma, or urinary reflux.
- Orchitis: an acute inflammation of the testis. The testis is painful and swollen. Generally occurs after an episode of bacterial or viral infections such as mumps, pneumonia, tuberculosis, or syphilis.

Congenital Problems

Cryptorchidism (undescended testes): failure of the testes to descend into the scrotal sac. Most common congenital testicular condition.

Acquired Problems

- Hydrocele: a nontender, fluid-filled mass.
- Spermatocele: a firm, sperm-containing, painless cyst of the epididymis.
- Varicocele: a dilation of the veins that drain the testes.
- Testicular torsion: a twisting of the spermatic cord. It is most commonly seen in males younger than age 20. The client experiences severe scrotal pain, swelling, nausea, and vomiting. Surgery is emergent.

Sexual Functioning

- Vasectomy: the bilateral surgical ligation of the vas deferens performed for the purpose of sterilization.
- Erectile dysfunction (ED): the inability to attain or maintain an erect penis that allows satisfactory sexual performance. ED is increasing in all segments of the sexually active male population. ED can result from a large number of factors.
  — Diabetes
  — Vascular disease
  — Side effects from medications
  — Result of surgery (prostatectomy)
  — Trauma
  — Chronic illness
  — Decreased gonadal hormone secretion
  — Stress
  — Difficulty in a relationship
  — Depression
  — Vascular disease (the most common cause)

The treatment for ED is based on the underlying cause.

Oral Drug Therapy

- sildenafil (Viagra)
- tadalafil (Cialis)
- vardenafil (Levitra)

HESI Hint

These drugs may potentiate the hypotensive effect of nitrates; they are contraindicated for individuals taking nitrates (such as nitroglycerin).

7 Movement, Coordination, and Sensory Input

Altered State of Consciousness
- Glasgow Coma Scale
  - Used to assess level of consciousness
  - Maximum score 15, minimum 3
  - A score of 7 or less = coma
  - Score of 3 to 4 = high mortality rate
  - Score of >8 = good prognosis
- Neurological vital signs
  - Pupil size (with sizing scale)
  - Limb movement (with scale)
  - Vital signs (blood pressure, temperature, pulse, respirations)

Nursing Assessment
- Assess for early S/S of changes in level of consciousness (LOC)
  - Decreasing LOC
  - Change in orientation
- Late signs
  - Cushing's triad
    - Widening pulse pressure
    - Slowing heart rate
    - Slowing respirations
  - Change in size, response of pupils, dilate on side of injury initially
  - Elevated temperature
- Assess for change in respiratory status
  - Cheyne-Stokes respiration
- Maintain airway: with decreasing LOC will need mechanical ventilation
- Prevent hypoxia
- Hyperventilate before suctioning
- Limit suctioning to 15 seconds
  - Keep airway free of secretions
  - Prevent aspiration

Treatment for Increased ICP
- ICP monitoring
  - Want ICP to be ≤15 mm Hg
- Hyperosmotic agents
  - 20% mannitol
- Steroids
  - Decadron
  - Solu-Medrol
- Barbiturates
- Prophylactic Dilantin
- Diuretics
  - Alternate with mannitol
- Avoid narcotics!

69

Which change in the status of a client being treated for increased ICP warrants immediate action by the nurse?
A. Urinary output changes from 20 to 50 mL/hr.
B. Arterial PCO₂ changes from 40 to 35 mm Hg.
C. Glasgow Coma Scale score changes from 5 to 7.
D. Pulse changes from 88 to 68 beats/min.

HESI Test Question Approach		
Positive?	YES	NO
Key Words		
Rephrase		
Rule Out Choices		
A	B	C	D

Head Injury

- Assessment
  — Changes in LOC
  — Signs of increased intracranial pressure (ICP)
  — Changes in VS
  — Headache
  — Vomiting
  — Pupillary changes
  — Seizure
  — Ataxia
  — Abnormal posturing (decerebrate or decorticate)

CSF Leakage

- Risk for meningitis with leakage
- May not see usual signs of increased ICP with leakage of CSF
- Drainage may come from nose (rhinorrhea) or ears (otorrhea)
- Altered cerebral perfusion related to ↑ ICP
  — MAP − ICP = CPP
  — Amount of blood flow from systemic circulation required to provide oxygen to the brain
  — Ideally CPP should be >70 mm Hg

Nursing Interventions

- Neurological assessment every 15 minutes
- Notify MD at *first* sign of deterioration
- Limit visitors
- Keep room quiet
- Prevent straining
- Keep HOB at 30 to 45 degrees
- Avoid neck flexion/straining
- Monitor I & O

The nurse is planning a class on stroke prevention for clients with hypertension. What information is most important to provide the clients in the class?

A. Salt restriction diet
B. Weight reduction
C. Medication compliance
D. Risk for stroke

<table>
<tr><td colspan="4">HESI Test Question Approach</td></tr>
<tr><td>Positive?</td><td></td><td>YES</td><td>NO</td></tr>
<tr><td colspan="4">Key Words</td></tr>
<tr><td colspan="4"></td></tr>
<tr><td colspan="4"></td></tr>
<tr><td colspan="4">Rephrase</td></tr>
<tr><td colspan="4"></td></tr>
<tr><td colspan="4"></td></tr>
<tr><td colspan="4">Rule Out Choices</td></tr>
<tr><td>A</td><td>B</td><td>C</td><td>D</td></tr>
</table>

STROKE (BRAIN ATTACK) OR CEREBROVASCULAR ACCIDENT

- Hemorrhage into brain tissue
- Ischemic clot
  — Thromboembolic
  — Embolic

Nursing Plans and Interventions

- Assess for S/S of increased ICP
- Assess verbal ability and plan care appropriate to client's ability to communicate
- Assess swallowing—prevent aspiration
- Assess for bowel and bladder control
- Assess functional abilities
  — Mobility
  — Activities of daily living (ADLs)
  — Elimination

Which client is best to assign to a graduate nurse being oriented to the neurological unit?

A. A head-injured client with a Glasgow Coma Scale score of 6
B. A client who develops autonomic dysreflexia following a T6 spinal cord injury
C. A client with multiple sclerosis who needs the first dose of interferon
D. A client suspected of having Guillain-Barré syndrome

<table>
<tr><td colspan="4">HESI Test Question Approach</td></tr>
<tr><td>Positive?</td><td></td><td>YES</td><td>NO</td></tr>
<tr><td colspan="4">Key Words</td></tr>
<tr><td colspan="4"></td></tr>
<tr><td colspan="4"></td></tr>
<tr><td colspan="4">Rephrase</td></tr>
<tr><td colspan="4"></td></tr>
<tr><td colspan="4"></td></tr>
<tr><td colspan="4">Rule Out Choices</td></tr>
<tr><td>A</td><td>B</td><td>C</td><td>D</td></tr>
</table>

PARKINSON'S DISEASE

- Triad of symptoms
- Rigidity
  — Masklike face
- Akinesia
  — Difficulty initiating and continuing movement
- Tremors
  — Resting tremors
  — Pill rolling

Nursing Plans and Interventions

- *Safety* is always a priority!
- Take medications with meals
- Change positions slowly to decrease postural hypotension
- Thicken liquids
- Soft foods
- Encourage activity and exercise

GUILLAIN-BARRÉ SYNDROME

- Usually occurs after an upper respiratory infection
- Ascending paralysis
- Rapid demyelination of the nerves
- Paralysis of respiratory system may occur quickly
- Prepare to intubate
- Treatment
  — Plasmapheresis over 10 to 15 days
  — IV high-dose immunoglobulin (Sandoglobulin) is effective as plasma exchange and has the advantage of immediate availability and greater safety. Clients receiving high-dose immunoglobulin need to be well hydrated and have adequate renal function.
  — Maintain patent airway
  — Reposition frequently
  — Impaired swallowing may need TPN
  — Supervise feedings

MULTIPLE SCLEROSIS

- Demyelination of the central nervous system (CNS) myelin
- Messages are garbled
- Messages are short-circuited from the brain to the CNS
- Disease is characterized by periods of remissions and exacerbations
- Assessment findings include:
  — Changes in visual field
  — Weaknesses in extremities
  — Numbness
  — Visual or swallowing difficulties
  — Unusual fatigue
  — Gait disturbances

Nursing Interventions

- Keep objects labeled
- Avoid quick changes in room lighting
- Provide assistive devices
- Thickened liquid

Parkinson's Disease Drug Therapy

- Dopaminergics
  — Levodopa (l-dopa, dopamine)
    - Blocks breakdown of levodopa to allow more levodopa to cross the blood-brain barrier
    - Avoid foods high in vitamin B_6 and high-protein foods
  — Levodopa-carbidopa (Sinemet, Parcopa [orally dissolving tablet])
    - Allows for less use of levodopa and helps decrease side effects
  — Bromocriptine mesylate (Parlodel)
    - Helps with motor fluctuations
  — Pergolide (Permax)
  — Pramipexole (Mirapex)
  — Ropinirole (Requip)
  — Amantadine (Symmetrel)
  — Apomorphine (Apokyn)
- Anticholinergics: treat tremors
  — Trihexyphenidyl (Artane)
  — Benztropine (Cogentin)
  — Biperiden (Akineton)
- Antihistamine
  — Diphenhydramine (Benadryl)
- Monoamine oxidase inhibitors
  — Selegiline (Eldepryl, Carbex)
  — Rasagiline (Azilect)
- Catechol-o-methyl transferase (COMT) inhibitors
  — Entacapone (Comtan)
  — Tolcapone (Tasmar)

MS Drug Therapy

- Focus on controlling symptoms
- Corticosteroids
  — ACTH, prednisone, methylprednisolone
- Immunomodulators
  — Interferon beta (Betaseron, Avonex, Rebif)
  — Glatiramer acetate (Copaxone)
- Immunosuppressants
  — Mitoxantrone (Novantrone)
- Cholinergics
  — Bethanechol (Urecholine)
  — Neostigmine (Prostigmin)
- Anticholinergics
  — Propantheline (Pro-Banthine)
  — Oxybutynin (Ditropan)
- Muscle relaxants
  — Diazepam (Valium)
  — Baclofen (Lioresal)
  — Dantrolene (Dantrium)
  — Tizanidine (Zanaflex)
- CNS stimulants
  — Pemoline (Cylert)
  — Methylphenidate (Ritalin)
  — Modafinil (Provigil)
- Antiviral/antiparkinsonian drugs
  — Symmetrel (Amantadine)

MYASTHENIA GRAVIS

- A chronic neuromuscular autoimmune disease
- Caused by loss of ACH receptors in the postsynaptic neurons at the neuromuscular junction
- ACH is necessary for muscles to contract
- Causes weakness and abnormal fatigue of voluntary muscles

Nursing Assessment

- Ocular muscle weakness
- Bulbar muscle weakness
- Skeletal muscle weakness
- Diagnosis
- Based upon clinical presentation
  — Muscle weakness
- Confirmed by testing response to anticholinesterase drugs
- Tensilon test—2 mg IV
- Medications
- Anticholinesterase agents
  — Try to achieve maximum strength and endurance
  — Blocks action of cholinesterase
  — Increase levels of ACH at junctions
  — Common medications
    - Mestinon
    - Prostigmin
  — Start with minimal doses
  — Onset 30 minutes
  — Duration 3 to 4 hours
  — Must take on time!
- Corticosteroids
  — Prednisone
- Immunosuppressive agents
  — Azathioprine (Imuran)
  — Cyclophosphamide (Cytoxan)

Types of Crisis

- Myasthenic
  — MEDICAL EMERGENCY!
  — Caused by undermedication or infection
  — Positive Tensilon test
  — Changes in VS, cyanosis, loss of cough and gag reflex, incontinence
  — May require intubation
- Cholinergic
  — Results from overmedication
  — Toxic levels of anticholinesterase medications
  — Symptoms: abdominal cramps, diarrhea, excessive pulmonary secretions
  — Negative Tensilon test

Nursing Interventions

- Coughing and deep breathing exercises
- Suction equipment at bedside
- Sit upright when eating and 1 hour after
- Keep chin downward when swallowing
- Plan activities carefully, weakness is greater at the end of the day

73

Spinal Cord Injury

- Injuries are classified by:
  - Extent of injury
  - Level of injury
  - Mechanism of injury
- Injuries are classified as complete or incomplete
- Transection/partial transection
- Rule of thumb:
  - Injury above C8 = quadriplegic
  - Injury below C8 = paraplegic

Nursing Assessment

- Start with the ABCs
- Determine quality of respiratory status
- Check neurological status
- Assess vital signs
- Hypotension and bradycardia occur in injuries above T6

Nursing Plans and Interventions

- Immobilize and stabilize!
- Keep neck and body in anatomical alignment
- Maintain patent airway
- Cervical injuries will be placed in skeletal traction
- High-dose corticosteroids are used to control edema during first 24 hours
- Spinal shock
- Flaccid paralysis
  - Complete loss of reflexes
  - Hypotension
  - Bradycardia
  - Bowel and bladder distention
- Reverse as quickly as possible

Autonomic Dysreflexia

- Medical emergency that occurs in clients with injuries at or above T6
- Exaggerated autonomic reflex response
- Usually triggered by bowel or bladder distention
- S/S: severe headache, $\uparrow$BP, bradycardia, and profuse sweating
- Elevate head of bed (while maintaining correct alignment), relieve bowel or bladder distention
- Rehabilitation
- Watch for paralytic ileus
  - Assess bowel sounds
- Kinetic bed to promote blood flow
- Antiembolic stockings
- Protect from skin breakdown
- Bowel and bladder training
  - Keeping bladder empty and urine dilute and acidic to help prevent urinary tract infection, a common cause of death after spinal cord injury

Which action by the unlicensed assistive personnel (UAP) requires immediate follow-up by the nurse?

A. Positions a client who is 12 hours post–above-knee amputation (AKA) with the residual limb elevated on a pillow

B. Assists a client with ambulation while the client uses a cane on the unaffected side

C. Accompanies a client who has lupus erythematosus to sit outside in the sun during a break

D. Helps a client with rheumatoid arthritis to the bathroom after the client receives Celebrex

HESI Test Question Approach			
Positive?		YES	NO
Key Words			
Rephrase			
Rule Out Choices			
A	B	C	D

Fractures
- Signs and Symptoms
- Pain, swelling, deformity of the extremity
- Discoloration, loss of functional ability
- Fracture evident on x-ray

Nursing Plans and Interventions
- Instruct on proper use of assistive devices
  — Assess for the 5Ps of neurovascular functioning
    • Pain, paresthesia, pulse, pallor, and paralysis
- Assess neurovascular area distal to injury
  — Skin color, temperature, sensation, capillary refill, mobility, pain, and pulses
- Intervention
  — Closed reduction
  — Open reduction
- Postreduction
  — Cast
  — Traction
  — External fixation
  — Splints
  — Orthoses (braces)

Joint Replacement
- Following surgery
  — Check circulation, sensation, and movement of extremity distal to replacement area
  — Keep body in proper alignment
  — Encourage fluid intake
  — Use of bedpan, commode chair
  — Coordinate rehabilitation process
- Discharge home
  — Safety
  — Accessibility
- Drugs
  — Anticoagulants
  — Analgesics
  — Parenteral antibiotics

Amputation
- Postoperative care will include:
- Monitoring surgical dressing for drainage
- Proper body alignment
- Elevate residual limb (stump) first 24 hours

75

- Do *not* elevate after 48 hours
- Provide passive range of motion (ROM) and encourage prone position periodically to decrease risk of contracture
- Proper stump bandaging to prepare for prosthesis
- Coordination of care with OT and PT

The nurse is assessing a client who is scheduled for surgical fixation of a compound fracture of the right ulna. Which finding should the nurse report to the healthcare provider?
A. Ecchymosis around the fracture site
B. Crepitus at the fracture site
C. Paresthesia distal to the fracture site
D. Diminished range of motion of the right arm

Musculoskeletal Problems

A postmenopausal woman who has a BMI of 18 is at the clinic for her annual well-woman's examination. Which teaching plan topic should the nurse prepare for this high-risk client?
A. Osteoporosis
B. Obesity
C. Anorexia
D. Breast cancer

Osteoporosis

- Risk factors
- Small postmenopausal females
- Diet low in calcium
- Excessive alcohol, tobacco, and caffeine
- Inactive lifestyle
- Low testosterone level in men

Nursing Assessment

- Dowager's hump
- Kyphosis of the dorsal spine
- Loss of height
- Pathological fractures
- Compression fracture of spine can occur

Nursing Plans and Interventions

- Keep bed in low position
- Provide adequate lighting
- Avoid using throw rugs

Amputation Drugs
- Analgesics
  — Phantom pain is *real*
- Antibiotics

HESI Test Question Approach		
Positive?	YES	NO
Key Words		
Rephrase		
Rule Out Choices		
A	B	C	D

HESI Test Question Approach		
Positive?	YES	NO
Key Words		
Rephrase		
Rule Out Choices		
A	B	C	D

Osteoporosis Drug Therapy
- Bisphosphonates
  — Alendronate (Fosamax)
  — Clodronate (Bonefos)
  — Etidronate (Didronel)
  — Ibandronate (Boniva)
  — Pamidronate (Aredia)
  — Risedronate (Actonel)
  — Tiludronate (Skelid)
- Selective estrogen receptor modulator
  — Raloxifene (Evista)
  — Teriparatide (Forteo)

- Provide assistance with ambulation
- Follow regular exercise program
- Diet high in vitamin D, protein, and calcium

Rheumatoid Arthritis
- Chronic, systemic, progressive deterioration of the connective tissue
- Etiology: unknown, believed to be autoimmune

Nursing Assessment
- Young to middle age
- More females than males
- Systemic with exacerbating and remissions
- Small joints first, then spreads
- Stiffness (may decrease with use)
- Decreased range of motion
- Joint pain
- Elevated erythrocyte sedimentation rate (ESR)
- Positive rheumatoid factor (RF) in 80% of clients
- Narrowed joint space

Nursing Plans and Interventions
- Drug therapy
  — High-dose ASA or NSAIDs
  — Systemic corticosteroids
  — Disease-modifying antirheumatic drugs (DMARDs)
    • Methotrexate (Rheumatrex)
    • Sulfasalazine (Azulfidine)
    • Hydroxychloroquine (Plaquenil)
    • Leflunomide (Arava)
- Heat and cold applications
- Weight management
- Rest and joint protection
- Use assistive devices
- Shower chair
- Canes, walkers
- Straight back chairs, elevated seats

Lupus Erythematosus
- Two classifications of lupus erythematosus
  — Discoid lupus erythematosus (DLE): Affects skin only
  — Systemic lupus erythematosus (SLE): More prevalent than DLE
- Major trigger factors
  — Sunlight
  — Infectious agents
  — Stress
  — Drugs
  — Pregnancy

Nursing Assessment
- DLE: scaly rash, butterfly rash over bridge of nose
- SLE: joint pain, fever, nephritis, pericarditis (Figure 7-1)
- Photosensitivity

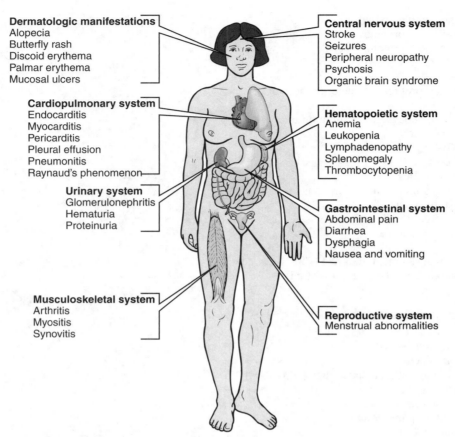

Dermatologic manifestations
Alopecia
Butterfly rash
Discoid erythema
Palmar erythema
Mucosal ulcers

Cardiopulmonary system
Endocarditis
Myocarditis
Pericarditis
Pleural effusion
Pneumonitis
Raynaud's phenomenon

Urinary system
Glomerulonephritis
Hematuria
Proteinuria

Musculoskeletal system
Arthritis
Myositis
Synovitis

Central nervous system
Stroke
Seizures
Peripheral neuropathy
Psychosis
Organic brain syndrome

Hematopoietic system
Anemia
Leukopenia
Lymphadenopathy
Splenomegaly
Thrombocytopenia

Gastrointestinal system
Abdominal pain
Diarrhea
Dysphagia
Nausea and vomiting

Reproductive system
Menstrual abnormalities

Figure 7-1   From Lewis, S., Heitkemper, M., Dirksen, S., O'Brien, P., & Bucher, L. (2007). *Medical-surgical nursing: Assessment and management of clinical problems* (7th ed.). St Louis: Mosby.

Nursing Plans and Interventions

■ Teaching
   — Drugs
   — Pain management
   — Disease process
   — Conservation of energy
   — Avoid exposure to ultraviolet rays
   — Avoid/reduce stress
   — Use mild soaps, creams for skin care
   — Use of steroids for joint inflammation
■ Therapeutic exercise and heat therapy
■ Marital and pregnancy counseling

Degenerative Joint Disease (Osteoarthritis)

■ Joint pain increases with activity
■ Morning stiffness
■ Crepitus
■ Limited movement
■ Joint enlargements

Nursing Plans and Interventions

■ Follow weight reduction diet
■ Excessive use of involved joint may accelerate degeneration
■ Use proper body mechanics

- Keep joints in functional position
- Hot and cold applications for pain and stiffness
- NSAIDs, opioid analgesics, and intraarticular corticosteroids

The nurse observes an elderly male client with glaucoma administer eye drops by tilting his head back, instilling each drop close to the inner canthus, and keeping his eye closed for 15 seconds. What action should the nurse implement first?

A. Ask the client if another family member is available to administer the drops

B. Review the correct steps of the procedure with the client

C. Administer the eye drops correctly in the other eye to demonstrate the technique

D. Discuss the importance of correct eye drop administration for persons with glaucoma

HESI Test Question Approach		
Positive?	YES	NO
Key Words		
Rephrase		
Rule Out Choices		
A	B	C	D

Glaucoma

- Primary open-angle glaucoma
  - Drainage channels become clogged
  - Decrease flow trabecular meshwork
- Primary closure-angle glaucoma
  - Bulging lens disrupts flow
- The silent thief of vision
- Normally painless
- Loss of peripheral vision
- May see halos around lights
- Diagnosed with eye examination
  - Tonometer to measure intraocular pressure

Nursing Plans and Interventions

- Key to treatment is:
  - ↓ Intraocular pressure
    - ↓ Aqueous humor production
    - ↑ Drainage of aqueous humor
  - Teach client and family proper eye drop instillation
  - Teach client how to avoid activities that can increase intraocular pressure

Collaborative Therapy

- Ambulatory/home care for open-angle glaucoma
  - Drug therapy
    - β-Adrenergic blockers
    - α-Adrenergic agonists
    - Cholinergic agents (miotics)
    - Carbonic anhydrase inhibitors
  - Surgical therapy
  - Argon laser trabeculoplasty (ALT)
  - Trabeculectomy with or without filtering implant
- Acute care for closure-angle glaucoma
  - Topical cholinergic agent
  - Hyperosmotic agent
  - Laser peripheral iridotomy
  - Surgical iridectomy

Glaucoma Drug Therapy

- β-Adrenergic blockers
  - Betaxolol (Betoptic)
  - Levobunolol (Betagan)
  - Metipranolol (OptiPranolol)
  - Timolol maleate (Timoptic, Istalol)
- α-Adrenergic agonists
  - Dipivefrin (Propine)
  - Epinephrine (Epifrin, Eppy, Gaucon, Epitrate, Epinal, Eppy/N)
  - Apraclonidine (Lopidine)
  - Brimonidine (Alphagan)
  - Latanoprost (Xalatan)
- Cholinergic agents (Miotics)
  - Carbachol (Isopto Carbachol)
  - Pilocarpine (Akarpine; Isopto Carpine, Pilocar, Pilopine, Piloptic, Pilostat)
- Carbonic anhydrase inhibitors
  - Systemic
    - Acetazolamide (Diamox)
    - Dichlorphenamide (Daranide)
    - Methazolamide (Neptazane)
  - Topical
    - Brinzolamide (Azopt)
    - Dorzolamide (Trusopt)

79

Cataracts

- Clouding or opacity of the lens
- Early signs
  — Blurred vision
  — Decreased color perception
- Late signs
  — Double vision
  — Clouded pupil

Nursing Plans and Interventions for Cataract Removal

- Preoperative
  — Assess medications being taken
  — Anticoagulants should be stopped before surgery
  — Teach how to instill eye drops
- Postoperative
  — Eye shield should be worn during sleeping hours
  — Avoid lifting >10 lb
  — Avoid lying on operative side
  — Report signs of increased intraocular pressure
    - Acute pain

The nurse is teaching an 86-year-old who has glaucoma and bilateral hearing loss. Which intervention should the nurse implement?
A. Maintain constant eye contact
B. Stand on the side unaffected by glaucoma
C. Speak in a lower tone of voice
D. Keep the environment dimly lit

Eye Trauma/Injury

- Trauma
  — Determine type of injury
  — Position client in sitting position to decrease intraocular pressure
  — Never attempt to remove embedded object
  — Irrigate eye if a chemical injury has occurred
- Detached retina
  — Described as curtain falling over visual field
  — Painless
  — May have black spots or floaters (indicates bleeding has occurred with detachment)
  — Surgical repair of retina
  — Keep eye patch over affected area

- Combination therapy
  — Timolol maleate and dorzolamide (Cosopt)
- Hyperosmolar agents
  — Glycerin liquid (Ophthalgan, Osmoglyn Oral)
  — Isosorbide solution (Ismotic)
  — Mannitol solution (Osmitrol)

HESI Test Question Approach			
Positive?		YES	NO
Key Words			
Rephrase			
Rule Out Choices			
A	B	C	D

Hearing Loss

- Conductive hearing loss
  - Sounds do not travel to the inner ear
  - May benefit from hearing aid
- Sensorineural hearing loss
  - Sound distorted from defect in inner ear
- Common causes
  - Infections
  - Ototoxic drugs
    - Gentamicin
    - Vancomycin
    - Lasix
  - Trauma
  - Aging process
- Assessment
  - Inability to hear whisper from 1 to 2 feet
  - Shouting in conversations
  - Turning head to favor one ear
- Loud volume on TV

8 Pediatric Nursing

The nurse directs the unlicensed assistive personnel (UAP) to play with a 4-year-old child on bed rest. Which activity should the nurse recommend?
A. Monopoly board game
B. Looking at picture books
C. Fifty-piece puzzle
D. Hand puppets

HESI Test Question Approach			
Positive?		YES	NO
Key Words			
Rephrase			
Rule Out Choices			
A	B	C	D

GROWTH AND DEVELOPMENT

- The five major developmental periods
  - Prenatal
  - Infancy
  - Early childhood
  - Middle childhood
  - Later childhood (pubescence and adolescence)
- The developmental theories most widely used in explaining child growth and development:
  - Freud's psychosexual stages
  - Erikson's stages of psychosocial development
  - Piaget's stages of cognitive development
  - Kohlberg's stages of moral development

Normal Growth and Development
Know norms for growth and development
- Toddlers (1-3 years)
  - Throws ball overhand at 18 months
  - Two- to three-word sentences at 2 years
  - Toilet training starts around 2 years
  - Toddlers are ritualistic
  - No concept of time
  - Frequent tantrums
- Preschool (3-5 years)
  - Rides tricycle at 3 years
  - Favorite word: *Why?*
  - Sentences of 5 to 8 words

HESI Hint
NCLEX Focus Questions
- Know norms for growth and development!
  - Birth weight doubles by 6 months, triples by 12 months
  - Plays "peek-a-boo" by 6 months
  - Sits upright without support by 8 months
  - Fine pincer grasp by 10 to 12 months (can pick up Cheerios)

- School age (6-12 years)
  — Each year gains 4 to 6 lb, grows 2 inches
  — Learns to tell time
  — Socialization with peers very important
- Adolescence (12-19 years)
  — Rapid growth second only to the first year of life
  — Secondary sex characteristics develop

Pain Assessment and Management
- Assessment is based upon verbal and nonverbal cues from child, and includes parents' information.
- Use appropriate pain scale
- Safety is a major priority for administering medication.
- Make sure dose is *safe* for age and weight.

Immunization Teaching
- Common cold does *not* contraindicate getting immunization unless fever >99° F
- Normal to have fever <102° F, redness and soreness at site 2 to 3 days after injection
- Call MD if high-pitched crying, seizures, or high fever occur
- Use acetaminophen orally

Communicable Diseases
- The incidence of common childhood communicable diseases has declined greatly since the advent of immunizations, but they do occur and nurses should be able to identify the infection.
  — Measles
  — Rubeola
  — Rubella
  — Roseola
  — Mumps
  — Pertussis
  — Chickenpox
  — Diphtheria
  — Erythema infectiosum (fifth disease)
- Treat fever from infection with acetaminophen not ASA (acetylsalicylic acid, aspirin).
- Isolation is required during the infectious phase of the infection.
- Teaching is the primary intervention for prevention of spread.
- Supportive measures are given while the disease runs its course.

Poisonings
- Frequent cause of childhood injury—teach poison-proof methods for the home.
- GI disturbance is a common symptom
- Burns of mouth, pharynx with caustic poisonings
- Identify poisonous agent quickly.
- Do the ABCs
- Teach parents to not make the child vomit because it may cause more damage
- Call Poison Control Center or 911, based on how the child is acting

HESI Hint
NCLEX Question Focus
- Use knowledge from the immunization chart: www.cdc.gov/vaccines/recs/schedules/
- Childhood immunization
  — *Example: What would be the vaccines the nurse would expect to be prescribed for a 2-month-old brought into the pediatrician's office for a well checkup? DTaP, HepB, HIB, IPV, and PCV*
  — *Example: Withhold MMR vaccine for person with history of anaphylactic reaction to neomycin or eggs.*

The nurse is performing an initial assessment of a 2-year-old child with suspected bacterial epiglottitis. What assessment is needed?

A. Use a tongue depressor to assess for erythema
B. Obtain a throat swab for culture and sensitivity
C. Observe for the presence of drooling
D. Measure pain using a FACES scale

HESI Test Question Approach			
Positive?		YES	NO
Key Words			
Rephrase			
Rule Out Choices			
A	B	C	D

RESPIRATORY DYSFUNCTION

- Respiratory dysfunction
  - Infection of the respiratory tract
  - Croup syndromes
  - Tuberculosis
  - Asthma
  - Cystic fibrosis

Respiratory Infections

- Nasopharyngitis
- Tonsillitis
  - May be viral or bacterial
  - Treatment important if related to streptococcal infection
  - Check prothrombin time (PT) and partial thromboplastin time (PTT) before surgery
  - Monitor for bleeding
  - Highest risk for bleeding is during first 24 hours and 5 to 10 days postoperative
- Otitis media
  - S/S: fever, pulling at ear
  - Discharge from ear
  - Administer antibiotics
  - Reduce temperature to prevent seizures
- Bacterial tracheitis
- Bronchitis
- Respiratory syncytial virus bronchiolitis
  - Isolate the child (contact isolation)
  - Monitor respiratory status
  - Antiviral agent (ribavirin aerosols)
  - Maintain patent airway
- Epiglottitis
  - S/S: high fever, sore throat, muffled voice, tripod position
  - IV antibiotics
  - Do not examine throat—may cause complete airway obstruction

Asthma

- The leading cause of chronic illness in children
- Allergies influence persistence and severity
- Complex disorder involving biochemical, immunologic, infections, endocrine and psychological factors.

HESI Hint
Respiratory Disorders

- Be familiar with normal values for respiratory and pulse rates for children.
- Know cardinal and other signs of respiratory distress.
- Respiratory failure will usually occur before cardiac failure.

85

Nursing Assessment and Interventions

- S/S: tight cough, expiratory wheezing, peak flow levels
- Monitor for respiratory distress, need for O_2 nebulizer therapy

Cystic Fibrosis (CF)

- Most frequently occurring inherited disease of Caucasian children
- Transmitted by an autosomal recessive gene
- Diagnosis of CF may be based on a number of criteria
  - Identification of CF mutations
  - Absence of pancreatic enzymes
  - Steatorrhea
  - Chronic pulmonary involvement
    - Prevent respiratory infections
- Positive newborn screening test
  - First sign may be meconium ileus at birth
  - High sweat chloride concentration (pilocarpine test or sweat test)
- Delayed growth—poor weight gain
- Pancreatic enzymes with each meal and snacks
- Fat-soluble vitamins
- Teach family percussion and postural drainage techniques

CARDIOVASCULAR DISORDERS

Congenital Heart Disorders

- May be classified as:
- Acyanotic: All have L to R shunt
  - Ventricular septal defect
  - Atrial septal defect
  - Patent ductus arteriosus
  - Coarctation of the aorta
  - Aortic stenosis
- Cyanotic:
  - Tetralogy of Fallot
  - Truncus arteriosus
  - Transposition of the great vessels

Nursing Interventions

- Maintain nutritional status, feeding should not last >30 min
- Plan frequent rest periods
- Administer digoxin, diuretics and angiotensin-converting enzyme (ACE) inhibitors as prescribed

Congestive Heart Failure

- Common complication of congenital heart disorders
- S/S: pedal edema, neck vein distention, cyanosis, grunting
- Monitor vital signs, elevate head of bed, O_2
- Digoxin, diuretics, and ACE inhibitors
- Weigh daily on same scale

For illustrations of cardiovascular disorders, see a textbook or an NCLEX Review Manual:

- *HESI Comprehensive Review for the NCLEX-RN Examination*
- *Mosby's Comprehensive Review of Nursing for NCLEX-RN Examination*
- *Saunders Comprehensive Review for the NCLEX-RN Examination*

Managing Digoxin Therapy in Children

- Hold in infants <100 beats/min, children <80 beats/min
- Do not skip or try to make up doses
- Give 1 to 2 hours before meals
- Watch for S/S of toxicity and teach parents
  - Vomiting, anorexia, diarrhea, muscle weakness, drowsiness

Rheumatic Fever

- Peaks in school-age children
- Most common cause of acquired heart disease
- Affects connective tissue
- S/S: sore throat, appears to be getting better, then fever develops along with rash, chorea, elevated erythrocyte sedimentation rate

Nursing Care Management

- Encourage compliance with drug regimens
  - Penicillin remains the drug of choice
  - Salicylates are used to control the inflammatory process and to reduce fever and discomfort.
  - Prednisone may be indicated in some patients with heart failure.
- Facilitate recovery from the illness
  - Bed rest or at least limited activity during the acute illness
- Provide emotional support

The nurse reviews the medication record of a 2-month-old and notes that the infant was given a scheduled dose of digoxin with a documented apical pulse of 76 beats/min. What action should the nurse take first?
A. Assess the current apical heart rate
B. Observe for the onset of diarrhea
C. Complete an adverse occurrence report
D. Determine the serum potassium level

HESI Test Question Approach			
Positive?		YES	NO
Key Words			
Rephrase			
Rule Out Choices			
A	B	C	D

A child with hydrocephalus is 1-day postoperative for revision of a ventriculoatrial shunt. Which finding is most important?
A. Increased blood pressure
B. Increased temperature
C. Increased serum glucose
D. Increased hematocrit

HESI Test Question Approach			
Positive?		YES	NO
Key Words			
Rephrase			
Rule Out Choices			
A	B	C	D

NEUROMUSCULAR DISORDERS

Down Syndrome

- Flat, broad nasal bridge; upward, outward slant of eyes
- Commonly associated problems
  - Cardiac defects
  - Delayed development
  - Respiratory problems

Cerebral Palsy (CP)

- Diagnosis made on evaluation of child
  - Persistent neonatal reflexes after 6 months
  - Spasticity
  - Scissoring of legs
  - Tight abductor muscles of hips
  - Tightening of heel cord
  - No parachute reflex
  - Prevent aspiration with feedings
  - phenytoin (Dilantin) for seizures
  - diazepam (Valium) for muscle spasms

Spina Bifida Occulta

- No sac present
- Suspect if tuft of hair at base of spine

Meningocele

- Contains only meninges and spinal fluid
- No nerves are in spinal sac

Myelomeningocele

- Sac contains spinal fluid, meninges, and nerves
- Will have sensory and motor defects
- Preoperative/postoperative care:
  - Monitor urine output
  - Watch for ↑ ICP
  - Keep sac free of stool/urine
  - Measure head circumference every 8 hours and check fontanels

Hydrocephalus

- Abnormal accumulation of cerebrospinal fluid (CSF)
- Symptoms
  - ↑ Intracranial pressure (ICP)
  - ↑ BP
  - ↓ Pulse
  - Changes in level of consciousness
  - Irritability and vomiting
- Interventions
  - Elevate head of bed
  - Seizure precautions
  - Prepare for shunt placement
    - Assess for shunt malfunctioning
    - Monitor for S/S of infection
  - Teaching related to shunt replacement

HESI Hint

- NCLEX-RN questions are likely to relate to supporting the child/parent to achieve the highest level of functioning.
  - Always evaluate mental age
  - Feed to back and side of mouth due to tongue thrust
  - Refer family to early intervention program

Seizures

- More common in children under 2 years
- Types of seizures
  - Generalized tonic/clonic
    - Grand mal seizure with loss of consciousness
    - Aura precedes seizure
    - Tonic phase: stiffness of body
    - Clonic phase: spasms and relaxation
    - Postictal phase: sleepy and disoriented
  - Petit mal
    - Momentary loss of consciousness, appears like daydreaming
    - Lasts 5 to 10 seconds

Nursing Plans and Interventions for Seizures

- Maintain patent airway
- Side rails up
- Pad side rails
- Administer anticonvulsants
- Teach family/client about medication

Bacterial Meningitis

- Usually caused by Streptococcus pneumoniae
- Signs and symptoms
  - Older children: include S/S of increased ICP, neck stiffness, + Kernig's sign, + Brudzinski's sign
  - Infants: classic signs absent, poor feeding, vomiting, irritability, bulging fontanels
- Diagnostic procedures include lumbar puncture for laboratory analysis
- Interventions
  - Isolate at least 24 hours
  - Administer antibiotics
  - Frequent VS and neurological checks
  - Increased ICP, muscle twitching, and changes in LOC
  - Measure head circumference daily
  - SIADH (syndrome of inappropriate antidiuretic hormone) occurs frequently
  - Fluid restrictions may be necessary

Reye Syndrome

- Etiology often, but *not always*, associated with aspirin use and influenza or varicella
- Rapidly progressing encephalopathy
- S/S: lethargy progressing to coma, vomiting, hypoglycemia
- Neurological checks, maintain airway
- Mannitol for ICP control
- Early diagnosis is important to improve client outcome

Anticonvulsants and Types of Seizures

- Phenobarbital
  - Generalized tonic-clonic
  - Partial
  - Status epilepticus
- Lamotrigine (Lamictal)
  - Absence
  - Myclonic
  - Partial
- Phenytoin (Dilantin)
  - Generalized tonic-clonic
  - Partial
  - Status epilepticus
- Valproic acid (Depakene)
  - Generalized tonic-clonic
  - Absence
  - Myoclonic
  - Partial
- Clonazepam (Klonopin)
  - Absence
  - Myoclonic
  - Infantile spasms
  - Partial
- Carbamazepine (Tegretol)
  - Generalized tonic-clonic
  - Partial

AGE	ORGANISM
Birth to 2 months	Enteric bacilli Group B streptococci
2 months to 12 years	*H. influenzae type b Streptococcus pneumoniae Neisseria meningitidis,* (meningococci)
12 years and older	*N. meningitidis S. pneumoniae*

Muscular Dystrophy (MD)

- Duchenne's MD
- Onset between ages 2 and 6 years
- Is the most severe and most common MD of childhood
- X-linked recessive disorder
- Diagnosis
  — Muscle biopsy muscle fibers degenerate and replaced by connective tissue and fat
  — Serum creatine phosphokinase (CK) levels are extremely high in the first 2 years of life before the onset
- Symptoms
  — Delayed walking
  — Frequent falls
  — Easily tires when walking
- Interventions
  — Exercise
  — Prevent falls
  — Assistive devices for ambulation

RENAL DISORDERS IN CHILDREN

Urinary Tract Infection (UTI)

- More common in girls
- Symptoms
  — Poor food intake
  — Strong-smelling urine
  — Fever
  — Pain with urination
- Interventions
  — Obtain urine culture before starting antibiotics
- Teach home care:
  — Finish all antibiotics
  — Avoid bubble baths
  — Increase intake of acidic fluids, such as apple or cranberry juice

Vesicoureteral Reflux

- Retrograde flow of urine into the ureters
- Symptoms
  — Recurrent UTIs
  — Common with neurogenic bladder
- Interventions
  — Teach to prevent UTI
  — Record output after catheterization
  — Maintain hydration

Acute Glomerulonephritis (AGN)

- Common features
  — Oliguria, hematuria, and proteinuria
  — Edema
  — Hypertension
  — Circulatory congestion
- Therapeutic management
  — Maintenance of fluid balance
  — Treatment of hypertension

90

- Assessment
  - Recent strep infection
  - Dark urine "iced tea"
  - Irritable and/or lethargic
- Interventions
  - VS every 4 hours
  - Daily weights
  - Low-sodium, low-potassium diet

Nephrotic Syndrome
Characterized by increased glomerular permeability to protein
- Management
  - Reducing excretion of protein
  - Reducing or preventing fluid retention
  - Preventing infection
- Assessment
  - Frothy urine
  - Massive proteinuria
  - Edema
  - Anorexia
- Intervention
  - Skin care
  - Administer medications
    - Diuretics
    - Corticosteroid therapy
    - Immunosuppressants
  - Small frequent feeding
- Discharge teaching
  - Daily weights
  - Side effects of meds
  - Prevent infections

Acute Renal Failure Management
- Treatment of the underlying cause
- Managing the complications of renal failure
- Providing supportive therapy

Abnormalities in Chronic Kidney Disease
- Waste product retention
- Water and sodium retention
- Hyperkalemia
- Acidosis
- Calcium and phosphorus disturbance
- Anemia
- Hypertension
- Growth disturbances

Home Dialysis
- Nursing interventions
- Educate the family about:
  - The disease, its implications, the therapeutic plan
  - Possible psychological effects
  - Treatment and technical aspects of the procedure
- Major concerns in kidney transplantation
  - Tissue matching
  - Prevention of rejection
- Psychological concerns
  - Self-image related to body changes from corticosteroid therapy

91

The nurse is planning care for an infant with a tracheoesophageal fistula. Which nursing diagnosis has the highest priority?

A. Infection, risk for
B. Injury, risk for
C. Nutrition, altered, less than
D. Aspiration, risk for

HESI Test Question Approach			
Positive?		YES	NO
Key Words			
Rephrase			
Rule Out Choices			
A	B	C	D

GASTROINTESTINAL DISORDERS

Nutritional Assessment

- Present nutritional status
- Body mass index
- Dietary history
- Past nutrition assessment
- Height
- Weight
- Head circumference
- Skinfold thickness
- Arm circumference
- Iron deficiency
  — $FeSO_4$ drops: use straw, give with orange juice, not with dairy foods

Diarrhea

- Worldwide leading cause of death in children <5 years of age
- Classified as acute or chronic
- Common problem for infants
- Nursing management goals
  — Fluid and electrolyte balance
  — Rehydration
  — Maintenance fluid therapy
  — Reintroduction of adequate diet
  — Do not give antidiarrheal agents
- Symptoms
  — Depressed sunken eyes
  — Weight loss
  — Decreased urine output

Cleft Lip or Cleft Palate

- Malformation of the face or oral cavity
- Initial closure of cleft lip is performed when infant weighs approximately 10 lb
- Closure of cleft palate at around 1 year
- Promote bonding
- Breck/Haberman feeder
- Maintain airway
- No straws, no spoons, only soft foods for cleft palate

Pyloric Stenosis
- Common in first-born males
- Vomiting becomes projectile around day 14 after birth

Perioperative Care of Client for Repair
Intussusception
- Telescoping of one part of intestine
- Emergency intervention is needed

Congenital Aganglionic Megacolon (Hirschsprung's Disease)
- Series of surgeries to correct
- Temporary colostomy

HEMATOLOGICAL DISORDERS

Iron Deficiency Anemia
- Common in infants, toddlers, and adolescent females
- Review Hgb norms for children
- Teach family about administering oral iron

Sickle Cell Anemia
- Autosomal recessive disorder
- Fetal Hgb does not sickle
- Hydration to promote hemodilution
- Symptoms
  — Crisis: Fever and pain
- Keep well hydrated
- Do not give supplemental iron
- Give folic acid orally

Hemophilia
- X-linked recessive disorder
- Interventions
  — Administer fresh frozen plasma
  — Apply pressure to even minor bleeds
- Increased risk for bleeding

METABOLIC AND ENDOCRINE DISORDERS

Phenylketonuria (PKU)
- Autosomal recessive disorder
- Newborn screening with Guthrie test
  — Done at birth and at 3 weeks
- Strict adherence to low-phenylalanine diet

Insulin-Dependent Diabetes Mellitus
- Common in school-age children
- Cognitive level and age should be considered when planning teaching
- Dietary teaching
- Exercise management
- Insulin administration

93

SKELETAL DISORDERS

Nursing Assessment

- Visible signs of fractures
- Obtain baseline pulses, color, movement, sensation, temperature, swelling, and pain
- Report any changes immediately

Traction

- Buck's traction
  — For knee immobilization
- Russell traction
  — For fracture of femur or lower leg
- Dunlap's traction
  — Can be skeletal or skin
- 90°/90° traction
- Provide appropriate toys, teach cast care to family, prevent cast soilage with diapering

Congenital Dislocated Hip

- Assessment
  — Positive Ortolani sign
  — Unequal fold of skin on buttocks
  — Limited abduction of hip
- Intervention
  — Apply Pavlik harness (worn 24 hours a day)
  — Surgical correction
- Postoperative intervention
  — Hip spica cast care

Scoliosis

- S-shaped curvature of the spine.
- Most common nontraumatic skeletal condition in children.
- Scoliosis affects both genders at any age, but it is most commonly seen in adolescents.

Juvenile Rheumatoid Arthritis (JRA)

- Juvenile rheumatoid arthritis is the most common arthritic condition of childhood.
- These inflammatory diseases involve the joints, connective tissues, and viscera.
- The exact cause is unknown, but infections and an autoimmune response have been implicated.
- Therapy consists of administration of medications, such as NSAIDs, methotrexate, or aspirin, along with exercise, heat application, and support of joints.

HESI Hint:

Special PKU formula
- Avoid meat, milk, dairy, and eggs
- Use: fruits, juices, cereal, bread, and starches

The LPN is assigned to care for a 3-year-old with Reye syndrome. The child's temperature is 102.4° F, and the LPN is preparing to administer aspirin PO. What action should the charge nurse implement?

A. Direct the LPN to assess the gag reflex and LOC.

B. Advise the LPN to wait until the fever is greater than 102.4° F.

C. Remind the LPN to hold all aspirin-containing medication.

D. Tell the LPN to notify the healthcare provider.

HESI Test Question Approach			
Positive?		YES	NO
Key Words			
Rephrase			
Rule Out Choices			
A	B	C	D

9 Maternal-Newborn Nursing

A 36-week gestational client is placed in the lithotomy position and suddenly complains of feeling breathless and light-headed, and exhibits marked pallor. What action should the nurse implement first?

A. Turn to a lateral position

B. Place in Trendelenburg position

C. Obtain vital signs and pulse oximeter

D. Initiate distraction techniques

HESI Test Question Approach			
Positive?		YES	NO
Key Words			
Rephrase			
Rule Out Choices			
A	B	C	D

- Assess for violence
  - Battering, emotional or physical abuse can begin with pregnancy
  - Assess for abuse in private, away from the male partner
  - The nurse needs to know
    - Local resources
    - How to determine safety of client
- Gravidity and parity
  - Gravida: number of times one has been pregnant regardless of outcome
  - Para: number of deliveries (not children) occurring after 20 weeks of gestation
    - Multiple births count as one
    - Pregnancy loss before 20 weeks counted as abortion but add 1 to gravidity
    - Fetal demise after 20 weeks is added to parity
- GTPAL equals number of
  - Term pregnancies
  - Preterm pregnancies
  - Abortions (elective or spontaneous)
  - Living children
- Gestation
  - Naegele's rule
    - Count back 3 months from date of last normal menstrual period
    - Add 1 year and 7 days
  - Example: If the last menstrual period was May 2, 2008, EDB would be February 9, 2009
- Fundal height
  - At 12 to 13 weeks: fundus rises out of symphysis
  - At 20 weeks: fundus at umbilicus
  - From 24 weeks to about 36 weeks: fundal height (measured in centimeters) from the symphysis is equal to number of weeks of gestation if it is a single pregnancy

- Psychological maternal changes
  - Ambivalence occurs early in pregnancy, even with planned pregnancy
  - Acceptance: occurs with the woman's readiness for the experience and her identification with the motherhood role.
  - Emotional lability refers to the frequent changes of emotional states or extremes in emotional states.

A female client has her suspected pregnancy confirmed. The client tells the nurse she had one pregnancy that she delivered at 39 weeks, twins that she delivered at 34 weeks, and a single gestation that she delivered at 35 weeks. Using the GTPAL notation, how should the nurse record the client's gravidity and parity?
A. 3-0-3-0-3
B. 3-1-1-1-3
C. 4-1-2-0-4
D. 4-2-1-0-3

HESI Test Question Approach			
Positive?		YES	NO
Key Words			
Rephrase			
Rule Out Choices			
A	B	C	D

The nurse is monitoring a client in the first stage of labor and identifies fetal heart rate (FHR) decelerations at the onset of each contraction and a return to the baseline after the contraction. What action should the nurse implement?
A. Discontinue the oxytocin infusion
B. Continue to monitor the FHR
C. Give a bolus of 750 mL D5LR
D. Insert a fetal scalp electrode

HESI Test Question Approach			
Positive?		YES	NO
Key Words			
Rephrase			
Rule Out Choices			
A	B	C	D

MATERNAL/FETAL MONITORING

- Time contractions
  - Frequency: from the beginning of one contraction to the beginning of the next contraction
  - Duration: length from the beginning to the end
  - Intensity: internal monitoring from 30 (mild) to 70 mm Hg (strong)
  - Resting tone/time: tension of uterine muscle between contractions and time between contractions
- Parameters of heart rates
  - Normal rate: 110-160 bpm
  - Tachycardia: >160 bpm
  - Bradycardia: <110 bpm

HESI Hint

External fetal monitoring is noninvasive and is achieved using a Toco transducer or Doppler ultrasonic transducer.

Internal fetal monitoring is invasive and requires rupturing of the membranes and attaching an electrode to the presenting part of the fetus.

- Nursing actions based on fetal heart rate, treat based on cause
  — Reassuring patterns
  — Accelerations
  — Nonreassuring patterns:
  — Late decelerations (always nonreassuring, even if not very "deep")

A woman who is in labor becomes nauseated, starts hiccupping, and tells her partner to leave her alone. The partner asks the nurse what he did to make this happen. How should the nurse respond?

A. "In active labor, it is quite common for women to react this way. It's nothing you did."

B. "I don't know what you did, but stop because she is quite sensitive right now."

C. "I'll come and examine her. This reaction is common during the transition phase of labor."

D. "Early labor can be very frustrating. I'm sure she doesn't mean to take it out on you."

HESI Test Question Approach		
Positive?	YES	NO
Key Words		
Rephrase		
Rule Out Choices		
A	B	C	D

Labor Progression

- Cervical dilation: stretching of cervical os from fingertip diameter to large enough to allow passage of infant (10 cm)
- Effacement: thinning and shortening of the cervix (0% to 100%)
- Station: location of the presenting part in relationship to the midpelvis or ischial spines, measured in centimeters above and below.
  — Station 0 = engaged
  — Station +2 = 2 cm below the level of the ischial spines
- Fetal presentation: part of the fetus that presents to the inlet
- Position: relationship of the point of reference (occiput sacrum, acromion) on the fetal presenting part to the mother's pelvis
  — LOA (left occiput anterior)—most common
- Lie: relationship of the long axis (spine) of the fetus to the long axis (spine) of the mother
  — Longitudinal: up and down
  — Transverse: perpendicular
  — Oblique: slanted
- Attitude: relationship of fetal parts to one another
  — Flexion: desired, so that smallest diameters are presented
  — Extension

True Labor

- Pain in lower back radiating to abdomen
- Regular, rhythmic contractions
- Increased intensity with ambulation
- Progressive cervical dilation and effacement

False Labor

- Discomfort localized to abdomen
- No lower back pain
- Contractions decrease in intensity and/or frequency with ambulation

The nurse performs a vaginal examination for a laboring client and determines the cervix is dilated 4 cm with 60% effacement, and the presenting part is at −2 station. Thirty minutes later, the client calls and says, "I think my water just broke." Which action has the highest priority?

A. Call the results to the healthcare provider
B. Evaluate the fetal heart rate
C. Help the client to the bathroom for hygiene
D. Perform the Nitrazine and fern tests

HESI Test Question Approach		
Positive?	YES	NO
Key Words		
Rephrase		
Rule Out Choices		
A	B	C	D

Types of Regional Blocks

- Pudendal block
  — Given in second stage
  — Has no effect on pain of uterine contractions
- Peridural (epidural or caudal) block
  — Given in first or second stage
  — Single dose or continuously
  — May prolong second stage
- Intradural (subarachnoid, spinal)
  — Given second stage
  — Rapid onset
  — Remain flat for 6 to 8 hours after delivery

Fundal Involution

- Immediately the fundus is several centimeters below the umbilicus
- Within 12 hours rises to the umbilicus
- Descends 1 cm (fingerbreadth) a day for 9 to 10 days, then fundus is below the symphysis pubis
- Should be midline and firm.

Teaching Points

- Change pads as needed and with voiding/defecation. Wipe front to back
- Good hand-washing technique
- Ice packs, sitz baths, peri bottle lavage, and topical anesthetic spray and pads
- Breast-feeding instructions
- Balance diet and fluid intake
- Rest/nap when baby sleeps
- Contraceptive use

Rh$_o$(D) Immune Globulin (RhoGAM)

- Given to Rh-negative women with possible exposure to Rh-positive blood
- Should have negative indirect Coombs' test
- Given IM within 72 hours after delivery
- Checked by two nurses (blood product)

Administration of Analgesic Medication
Drugs Used During Labor

- Fentanyl (Sublimaze)
- Morphine sulphate (MS Contin)
- Butorphanol tartrate (Stadol)
- Nalbuphine (Nubain)
- Dilaudid

Rubella Vaccine
- Given subcutaneously to nonimmune client before discharge from hospital
- May breastfeed
- Do not give if client or family member is immuno-compromised
- Avoid pregnancy for 2 to 3 months (teach contraception)

A client who is 72 hours postcesarean section is preparing to go home. She shares that she cannot get the baby's diaper on "right." Which action should the nurse implement?
A. Demonstrate how to correctly diaper the baby
B. Observe the client diapering the baby while offering praise and hints
C. Call the social worker for long-term follow-up
D. Reassure the client that she knows how to take care of her baby

HESI Test Question Approach			
Positive?		YES	NO
Key Words			
Rephrase			
Rule Out Choices			
A	B	C	D

Four births will occur at once. Which birth should the nursery charge nurse assign a newly licensed nurse as her first solo birth and admission?
A. G1 P0 at 39 weeks who will give birth vaginally after a 15-hour induced labor. The mother has been on magnesium sulfate for preeclampsia throughout the labor.
B. G5 P4 at 38 weeks who will give birth vaginally after a 5-hour unmedicated labor. Mild to moderate variable decelerations have been occurring for the last 15 minutes.
C. G3 P1 at 34 weeks who will give birth by cesarean section for a nonreassuring fetal heart rate pattern. The client has a history of cocaine use and has symptoms of abruptio placentae.
D. G2 P1 at 42 weeks who will give birth vaginally after induced labor. The client has been pushing for 2 hours and forceps will be used.

HESI Test Question Approach			
Positive?		YES	NO
Key Words			
Rephrase			
Rule Out Choices			
A	B	C	D

A 33-week-gestational woman who is diagnosed with pregnancy-induced hypertension (PIH) is admitted to the labor and delivery area. She is obviously nervous and expresses concern for the health of her baby. How should the nurse respond?
A. "You have the best doctor on the staff, so don't worry about a thing."
B. "Your anxiety is contributing to your condition and may be the reason for your admission."
C. "This is a minor problem that is easily controlled, and everything will be all right."
D. "As I assess you and your baby, I will explain the plan for your care and answer your questions."

HESI Test Question Approach			
Positive?		YES	NO
Key Words			
Rephrase			
Rule Out Choices			
A	B	C	D

Chronic Hypertension

- Hypertension and/or proteinuria in pregnant woman with chronic hypertension before 20 weeks of gestation and persistent after 12 weeks postpartum

Superimposed Preeclampsia or Eclampsia

- Development of preeclampsia or eclampsia in woman with chronic hypertension before 20 weeks of gestation

Preeclampsia/Eclampsia

HELLP syndrome: extremely severe form of gestational hypertension: **H**emolysis, **E**levated **L**iver Enzymes, **L**ow **P**latelets

- Preeclampsia symptoms
  - BP
    - Mild: 30 mm Hg systolic and/or 15 mm Hg diastolic over baseline
    - Severe: Same (some sources say 160/110 mm Hg × 2 or more)
  - Protein
    - Mild: >1+
    - Severe: 3+ to 4+
  - Edema
    - Mild: Eyes, face, fingers
    - Severe: Generalized edema
  - Deep tendon reflexes (DTRs)
    - Mild: 3+
    - Severe: 3+ or more and clonus
  - Central nervous system (CNS) symptoms
    - Mild: Headache, irritability
    - Severe: Severe headache, visual disturbances
  - Other
    - Weight gain >2 lb/week
    - Oliguria (<100 mL/4 hr); epigastric pain related to liver enlargement
    - Elevated serum creatinine, thrombocytopenia, marked SGOT elevation

Nursing Interventions: Preeclampsia

- Control stimulation in room
- Explain procedures
- Maintain IV (16 to 18 g venocatheter)
- Monitor BP every 15 to 30 minutes and DTRs and urine for protein every 1 hour
- Administer magnesium sulfate as prescribed
- Monitor magnesium levels and signs of toxicity (urinary output <30 mL/hr, R <12, DTRs absent, deceleration of FHR, bradycardia)

Nursing Interventions: Eclampsia (seizures)

- Stay with client
- Turn client to side
- Do not attempt to force objects into client's mouth
- Administer O$_2$ and have suction available
- Give magnesium sulfate as prescribed

HESI Hint

Magnesium sulfate is *not* an antihypertensive; it is used to prevent/control seizure. Withhold if any of the following is present:

- R <12 breaths/min
- Absent deep tendon reflexes (DTRs)
- Urine output <30 mL/hr

HESI Hint

Remember that seizures can occur postpartum.

Gestational Diabetes

Screening

■ Recommendations for glucose screening for all pregnant women
   — 1-hour glucose screen between 24 and 26 weeks

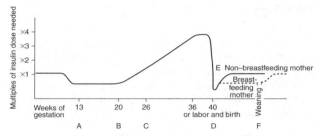

Figure 9-1   From Lowdermilk, D., & Perry, S. (2007). *Maternity and women's health care* (9th ed.). St Louis: Mosby.

A client who has gestational diabetes asks the nurse to explain the reason why her baby is at risk for macrosomia. Which explanation should the nurse offer?
A. The placenta receives decreased maternal blood flow during pregnancy because of vascular constriction.
B. The fetus secretes insulin in response to maternal hyperglycemia, causing weight gain and growth.
C. Infants of diabetic mothers are postmature, which allows the fetus extra time to grow.
D. Rapid fetal growth contributes to congenital anomalies, which are more common in infants of diabetic mothers.

HESI Test Question Approach			
Positive?		YES	NO
Key Words			
Rephrase			
Rule Out Choices			
A	B	C	D

Preterm Labor (PTL)

■ Signs and symptoms of PTL
   — More than five contractions in an hour; menstrual-like cramps
   — Low, dull backache
   — Pelvic pressure
   — Increase/change in vaginal discharge
   — Leaking or gush of amniotic fluid

Tocolytics and Their Administration

The medications used for cessation of uterine contractions include:
■ Ritodrine (Yutopar)
   — Side effects
      • Nervousness and tremulousness
      • Headache
      • N/V, diarrhea and epigastric pain
   — Adverse effects
      • Tachycardia
      • Chest pain with pulmonary edema
      • Low K^+ and hyperglycemia

HESI Hint

Betamethasone (Celestone) is used in PTL to enhance surfactant production and fetal lung maturity if fetus is <35 weeks of gestation.

— Nursing interventions
  • Maternal ECG and lab tests
  • Cardiac and fetal monitoring
  • VS every 15 minutes
— Antidotes
  • Propranolol (Inderal)
■ Terbutaline (Brethine)
— Side effects
  • Nervousness and tremulousness
  • Headache
  • N/V, diarrhea and epigastric pain
— Adverse effects
  • Tachycardia
  • Chest pain with pulmonary edema
  • Low K^+ and hyperglycemia
— Nursing interventions
  • Maternal pulse not >140 bpm
  • FHR not >180 bpm
  • Monitor I & O
  • Check weight daily
— Antidotes
  • Propranolol (Inderal)
■ Magnesium sulfate
— Side effects
  • CNS depression
  • Slowed respirations
  • Decreased DTRs
— Adverse effects
  • Decreased urine output
  • Pulmonary edema
— Nursing interventions
  • Hold if R <12/min
  • Urine output <100 mL/4 hr
  • Absent DTRs
  • Monitor serum magnesium levels
— Antidote
  • Calcium gluconate
■ Additional drugs used to decrease contractions
— Indomethacin (Indocin)
— Nifedipine (Procardia)

A client at 15 weeks of gestation is admitted for an inevitable abortion. Thirty minutes after returning from surgery, her vital signs are stable. Which intervention has the highest priority?

A. Ask the client if she would like to talk about losing her baby.

B. Place cold cabbage leaves on the client's breasts to decrease breast engorgement.

C. Send a referral to the grief counselor for at-home follow-up

D. Confirm the client's Rh and Coombs' status and administer RhoGAM if indicated.

HESI Hint
Insulin
Generally, oral hypoglycemics are not used in pregnancy because they cross the placenta. Insulin is used because it does not cross the placenta.

Only regular insulin is used during labor because it is short acting, which makes it easier to maintain the mother's glucose level at 60 to 100 mg/dL.

HESI Hint
If abruption or previa is suspected or confirmed, *no* abdominal or vaginal manipulation such as
■ Leopold's maneuvers
■ Vaginal examinations
■ Internal monitor (especially if previa)
■ Rectal examinations/enemas/suppositories

HESI Test Question Approach		
Positive?	YES	NO
Key Words		
Rephrase		
Rule Out Choices		
A	B	C	D

Miscarriage

- Assessment
  - Vaginal bleeding with a gestational age of 20 weeks or less
  - Uterine cramping, backache, and pelvic pressure
  - Maybe symptoms of shock
  - Assess client/family emotional status, needs, and support
- Interventions
  - Monitor VS, LOC, and amount of bleeding
  - Prepare client to receive IV fluids and/or blood
  - If client Rh negative, give RhoGAM

Incompetent Cervix

Incompetent cervix (recurrent premature dilation of the cervix) is defined as passive and painless dilation of the cervix during the second trimester.

- Conservative management
  - Bed rest
  - Hydration
  - Tocolysis (inhibition of uterine contractions)
- A cervical cerclage may be performed.
  - McDonald cerclage: a band of homologous fascia or nonabsorbable ribbon (Mersilene) may be placed around the cervix beneath the mucosa to constrict the internal os of the cervix.
  - A cerclage procedure can be classified according to time, or whether it is elective (prophylactic), urgent, or emergent.

Ectopic Pregnancy

- Assessment
  - Missed period but early signs of pregnancy absent
  - Positive pregnancy test
  - Rupture
    - Sharp unilateral pelvic pain
    - Vaginal bleeding
    - Referred shoulder pain
    - Syncope can lead to shock
- Interventions
  - Monitor hemodynamic status
  - Prepare client for surgery and IV fluid administration including blood.

Abruptio Placentae and Placenta Previa

- Abruptio placentae
  - Concealed or overt bleeding
  - Uterine tone ranges from tense without relaxation to tense and boardlike
  - Persistently painful
  - Abnormal fetal heart rate (the more area abrupted, the worse the FHR)
- Placenta previa
  - Bright red vaginal bleeding
  - Soft uterine tone
  - Painless
  - FHR is normal unless bleeding is severe and mother becomes hypovolemic

105

Disseminated Intravascular Coagulation

- Risk factors for DIC in pregnancy
  — Fetal demise
  — Infection/sepsis
  — Pregnancy-induced hypertension (preeclampsia)
  — Abruptio placentae

Dystocia

- A difficult birth resulting from problems of the "5 Ps" (powers, passage, passenger, psyche, and/or position); that is, a lack of progress in cervical dilation, delay in fetal descent, or change in uterine contraction characteristics suggest dystocia.

Postpartum Infections

- Perineal infections
- Endometritis
- Parametritis
- Peritonitis
- Mastitis
- Deep vein thrombosis
- Cystitis
- Pyelonephritis
- HIV, hepatitis, other STIs

The nurse receives shift reports on four postpartum clients. Which client should the nurse assess first?
A. G3 P3, 7 hours after forceps delivery, who is complaining of pain and perineal pressure unrelieved by analgesics
B. G1 P1, 8 hours after cesarean delivery who is receiving IV Pitocin and complaining of cramping with increased lochia when sitting
C. G2 P2, 5 hours after vaginal delivery, complaining of abdominal pain when the infant breastfeeds
D. G7 P6, 6 hours after vaginal delivery of twins, who reports saturating one pad in a 3-hour period

Which nursing action has the highest priority for an infant immediately after birth?
A. Place the infant's head in the "sniff" position and give oxygen via face mask
B. Perform a bedside glucose test and feed the infant glucose water as needed
C. Assess the heart rate and perform chest compressions if rate is less than 60 bpm
D. Dry the infant and place under a radiant warmer or skin-to-skin with the mother

HESI Test Question Approach			
Positive?		YES	NO
Key Words			
Rephrase			
Rule Out Choices			
A	B	C	D

HESI Test Question Approach			
Positive?		YES	NO
Key Words			
Rephrase			
Rule Out Choices			
A	B	C	D

Newborn Parameters (approximate)

- Length: 18 to 22 inches; Weight: 5.5 to 9.5 lb
- Head circumference: 13.2 to 14 inches
- Head should be one-fourth of the body length
- Sutures are palpable with fontanels
- Fontanel closure
  — Anterior: by 18 months
  — Posterior: 6 to 8 weeks
- Umbilical cord should have three vessels—two arteries and one vein
- Extremities should be flexed
- Major gluteal folds even
- Creases on soles of feet
- Ortolani's sign and Barlow's sign for developmental dysplasia of the hip
- Pulses palpable (radial, brachial, femoral)

Nursing Actions

- Keep the newborn warm.
- Suction the airway as necessary
- Observe for respiratory distress
- Normal or physiological jaundice appears after the first 24 hours in full-term newborns
- Pathological jaundice occurs before this time and may indicate early hemolysis of red blood cells
- Assess the H&H and blood glucose levels.
- Weigh daily.
- Monitor intake and output; weigh diapers if necessary (1 g = 1 mL of urine).
- Monitor the temperature.
- Observe for any cracks in the skin.
- Administer eye medication within 1 hour after birth.
- Provide cord care.
- Provide circumcision care. Teach the client how to care for circumcision site.
- Position the newborn on the right side after feeding; however, the side-lying position is not recommended for sleep because this position makes it easy for the newborn to roll to the prone position
- Observe for normal stool and the passage of meconium.
- Test the newborn's reflexes.

Reflexes Exhibited and Age Reflexes Disappear

- Sucking or rooting: 3 to 4 months
- Moro: 3 to 4 months
- Tonic neck or fencing: 3 to 4 months
- Babinski's sign: 1 year to 18 months
- Palmar-plantar grasp: 8 months
- Stepping or walking: 3 to 4 months

MAJOR NEWBORN COMPLICATIONS

Respiratory Distress Syndrome

- Caused inability to produce surfactant
- Resulting in hypoxia and acidosis

Meconium Aspiration Syndrome

- Fetal distress increases intestinal peristalsis
- Releasing meconium into the amniotic fluid

Newborn Vital Signs

- Heart rate (resting): 100 to 160 beats/min (apical) by auscultating at the fourth intercostal space for 1 full minute
- Respirations: 30 to 60 breaths/min for 1 full minute
- Axillary temperature: 97.9° F to 98.6° F
- Blood pressure: 73/55 mm Hg

Hypoglycemia

Low level of glucose in the blood
- <40 mg/dL in the first 72 hours of life
- <45 mg/dL after the first 3 days of life

Normal blood glucose level
- 40 to 60 mg/dL in a 1-day-old newborn
- 50 to 90 mg/dL in a newborn older than 1 day.

Retinopathy of Prematurity

- Vascular disorder of retina
- Caused by the use of oxygen (>30 days)

Hyperbilirubinemia

- Elevated serum levels >12 mg/dL
- Prevention of kernicterus, which results in permanent neurological damage
- Jaundice starts at the head, spreads to the chest, abdomen, arms, legs, hands and feet
- Phototherapy is the use of fluorescent lights to reduce serum bilirubin levels
- Possible adverse effects: eye damage, dehydration, or sensory deprivation
- Expose as much of the skin as possible but cover the genital area
- Cover the eyes with eye shields
- Monitor skin temperature closely
- Increase fluids to compensate for water loss
- Expect loose green stools and green urine
- Monitor the newborn's skin color
- Reposition every 2 hours
- Provide stimulation
- After treatment, continue monitoring for signs of rebound hyperbilirubinemia

Erythroblastosis Fetalis

- Is the destruction of red blood cells that results from an antigen-antibody reaction
- Is characterized by hemolytic anemia or hyperbilirubinemia.
- Exchange of fetal and maternal blood occurs at birth Antibodies are harmless to the mother, but cause fetal hemolysis
- Administer Rho(D) immune globulin
- The newborn's blood is replaced with Rh-negative blood to stop the destruction of the newborn's red blood cells
- The Rh-negative blood is replaced with the newborn's own blood gradually.

Sepsis

- The presence of bacteria in the blood

TORCH Infections

- Infections that are caused by one of the following:
  - Toxoplasmosis
  - Other infections such as gonorrhea, syphilis, varicella, hepatitis B, HIV, or human parvovirus B19
  - Rubella
  - Cytomegalovirus
  - Herpes simplex virus

Addicted Newborn

- Passive addiction to drugs that have passed through the placenta

Fetal Alcohol Syndrome

- Caused by maternal alcohol use during pregnancy
- Causes mental and physical retardation

Newborn of a Mother with HIV

- Monitor antibody closely throughout pregnancy.

Newborn of a Diabetic Mother

- Infant born to mother with insulin-dependent diabetes or gestational diabetes
- Hypoglycemia, hyperbilirubinemia, respiratory distress syndrome, hypocalcemia, birth trauma, and congenital anomalies may be present.

A pregnant client tells the nurse that she smokes only a few cigarettes a day. What information should the nurse provide the client about the effects of smoking during pregnancy?

A. Smoking causes vasoconstriction and decreases placental perfusion.

B. Smoking decreases the L:S ratio, contributing to lung immaturity.

C. Smoking causes vasodilation and increased fluid overload for the fetus.

D. Smoking during pregnancy places the fetus at risk for lung cancer.

HESI Test Question Approach		
Positive?	YES	NO
Key Words		
Rephrase		
Rule Out Choices		
A	B	C	D

10 Mental Health Nursing

NURSE-CLIENT RELATIONSHIP

The goal of the nurse-client relationship is to help the client to develop problem-solving coping mechanisms.

THERAPEUTIC COMMUNICATION

- Is both verbal and nonverbal expression
- Is goal-directed
- Includes appropriateness, efficiency, flexibility, and feedback

MENTAL HEALTH

- A lifelong process
- Successful adjustment to changing environments (internal and external)

MENTAL HEALTH ILLNESS

- A loss of the ability to respond to the environment in accord with oneself and society.

A female client who just learned that she has breast cancer told her family that the biopsy was negative. What action should the nurse take?
A. Remind the client that the results were positive
B. Ask the client to restate what the healthcare provider told her
C. Talk to the family about the client's need for family support
D. Encourage the client to talk to the nurse about her fears

COPING AND DEFENSE MECHANISMS

- Efforts to decrease anxiety
- Can be constructive or destructive
- Coping is related to problem solving
- Defense is related to protecting oneself

HESI Hint

When a client discloses information to the nurse and then asks the nurse to avoid telling anyone….

The best response is to explain to the client that "information that is relevant to your treatment plan must be shared with the treatment team," especially if the client has thoughts of harm to self or others.

HESI Test Question Approach		
Positive?	YES	NO
Key Words		
Rephrase		
Rule Out Choices		
A	B	C	D

THERAPEUTIC TREATMENT MODALITIES

- Milieu therapy: The physical and social environment in which the client is receiving treatment
- Interpersonal psychotherapy: uses a therapeutic relationship to modify the client's feelings, attitudes, and behaviors
- Behavior therapy: Many forms and is used to change client behaviors
- Cognitive therapy: directive, time-limited approach

The nurse is facilitating a support group about stress management. During the initial phase, a female group member states that she can help the group more because she has a master's degree. How should the nurse respond?
A. Restate the purpose of the support group sessions
B. Ask the group to identify various stressful problems
C. Obtain ideas from the members about strategies for stressful situations
D. Conclude the meeting and evaluate the session

HESI Test Question Approach			
Positive?		YES	NO
Key Words			
Rephrase			
Rule Out Choices			
A	B	C	D

Group Therapy

- Involves a therapist and 5-8 members
- Provides feedback and support for the individual goals of each member
- Group therapy models
  - Psychoanalytical
  - Transactional analysis
  - Rogerian therapy
  - Gestalt therapy
- Interpersonal group therapy
- Self-help or support groups
- Family therapy
  - The member with the presenting symptoms indicates the presence of problems in the entire family.
  - A change in one member will bring about changes in other members.

Stages of Group Development

- Initial stage: superficial communication
- Working stage: real work is done by group.
- Termination stage: provides opportunity to learn to deal with letting go.

The nurse takes a group of mental health clients to a baseball game. During the game, a male client begins to complain of shortness of breath and dizziness. Which intervention should the nurse implement first?

A. Send the client back to the unit
B. Ask for a description of his feelings
C. Escort the client to a quiet area
D. Inquire about what is most stressful

HESI Test Question Approach			
Positive?		YES	NO
Key Words			
Rephrase			
Rule Out Choices			
A	B	C	D

ANXIETY

Anxiety is a normal subjective experience that includes feeling of apprehension, uneasiness, uncertainty, or dread.

Types of Anxiety

- Mild: tension of everyday life
- Moderate: immediate concerns
- Severe: feeling that something bad is about to happen
- Panic: terror and a sense of impending doom

Nursing Interventions

- Decrease stimuli in the environment
- Provide a calm quiet environment

DISORDERS

Generalized Anxiety Disorder

- An unrealistic anxiety about everyday worries
- Panic disorders produce a sudden feeling of intense apprehension.

Posttraumatic Stress Disorder

- Reexperience of traumatic event
- Recurrent and intrusive dreams or flashbacks

Phobias

- Irrational fear of an object, activity, or situation
- Client may recognize it as unreasonable
- Associated with panic level anxiety
- Defense mechanisms used include repression and displacement

The nurse is planning to teach a male client strategies for coping with his anxiety. The nurse finds him in his room compulsively washing his hands. What action should the nurse take next?
A. Teach alternatives as he washes his hands
B. Ask him to stop his hand washing immediately
C. Allow him to finish hand washing before teaching
D. Ask what precipitated the hand washing

HESI Test Question Approach			
Positive?		YES	NO
Key Words			
Rephrase			
Rule Out Choices			
A	B	C	D

Obsessive-Compulsive Disorder
- Obsessions: Persistently intrusive thoughts
- Compulsions: repetitive behaviors designed to divert unacceptable thought and decrease anxiety

Antianxiety or Anxiolytic Medications
- Antianxiety medications depress the CNS. Benzodiazepines have anxiety-reducing (anxiolytic), sedative-hypnotic, muscle-relaxing, and anticonvulsant actions.
- Flumazenil (Romazicon), a benzodiazepine antagonist administered intravenously, reverses benzodiazepine intoxication in 5 minutes.

Somatoform Disorders
Persistent worry or complaints regarding physical illness without physical findings.
- Types of somatoform disorders
  — Conversion disorder
  — Hypochondriasis
  — Somatization disorders

While the nurse is talking to a client who has a dissociative identity disorder, the client begins to dissociate during the interaction. Which action should the nurse implement?
A. Escort the client to art therapy group
B. Call the client by name
C. Talk about stressful feelings
D. Move to another setting

HESI Test Question Approach			
Positive?		YES	NO
Key Words			
Rephrase			
Rule Out Choices			
A	B	C	D

Dissociative Disorders

It is associated with exposure to an extremely traumatic event.

- Dissociative amnesia: one or more episodes of inability to recall important personal information, usually of a traumatic nature
- Dissociative fugue: a sudden, unexpected travel away from home, with an inability to recall one's past.
- Dissociative identity disorder: two or more distinct identities and at least two of these identities recurrently take control.
- Depersonalization disorder: persistent or recurrent episodes of feelings of detachment from one's self.

PERSONALITY DISORDERS

- Inflexible maladaptive behavior patterns
- In touch with reality
- Lack of insight into his or her behavior
- Forms of acting out include:
  — Yelling and swearing
  — Cutting own skin
  — Manipulation
  — Substance abuse
  — Promiscuous sexual behaviors
  — Suicide attempts

Cluster A (Odd and Eccentric)
- Paranoid
- Schizoid
- Schizotypal

Cluster B (Emotional and Dramatic)
- Antisocial
- Borderline
- Histrionic
- Narcissistic

Cluster C (Anxious and Tense)
- Avoidant
- Dependent
- Obsessive-compulsive

A female client who has borderline personality disorder returns after a weekend pass with lacerations to both wrists. The client whines and complains to the nurse during the dressing change. How should the nurse respond?
A. Distant
B. Concerned
C. Matter-of-fact
D. Empathetic

HESI Test Question Approach			
Positive?		YES	NO
Key Words			
Rephrase			
Rule Out Choices			
A	B	C	D

EATING DISORDERS

Compulsive Overeating

- Bingelike overeating without purging
- Lack of control over food consumption

Anorexia Nervosa

- Onset is often associated with a stressful event.
- Death can occur from starvation, suicide, cardiomyopathies, or electrolyte imbalance.
- The client experiences an altered body image.

Bulimia Nervosa

Binge-purge syndrome: Eating binges followed by purging behaviors.

A client with bulimia is admitted to the mental health unit. What intervention is most important for the nurse to include in the initial treatment plan?
A. Observe client after meals for vomiting
B. Assess daily weight and vital signs
C. Monitor serum potassium and calcium
D. Provide a structured environment at mealtime

MOOD DISORDERS

Depression/Suicide

Purpose

Antidepressants have been approved for depression, phobias, eating disorders and anxiety disorders.

Monoamine Oxidase Inhibitors (MAOIs)

- Inhibit the enzyme monoamine oxidase, which is present in the brain, blood platelets, liver, spleen, and kidneys.
- Clients who have depression and have not responded to other antidepressant therapies, including electroconvulsive therapy, are given MAOIs.
- Concurrent use with amphetamines, antidepressants, dopamine, epinephrine, guanethidine, levodopa, methyldopa, nasal decongestants, norepinephrine, reserpine, tyramine-containing foods, or vasoconstrictors may cause hypertensive crisis.
- Concurrent use with opioid analgesics may cause hypertension or hypotension, coma, or seizures.

Bipolar Disorder

- Characterized by episodes of mania and depression with periods of normal mood and activity in between
- Lithium carbonate: medication of choice can be toxic and requires regular monitoring of serum lithium levels
- Other medications:
  — divalproex (Valproate)
  — olanzapine (Zyprexa)
  — carbamazepine (Tegretol)

HESI Test Question Approach			
Positive?		YES	NO
Key Words			
Rephrase			
Rule Out Choices			
A	B	C	D

Nursing Implications and Client Education

Selective Serotonin Reuptake Inhibitors (SSRIs)

- Inhibit serotonin uptake

Tricyclic Antidepressants

- Blocks the reuptake of norepinephrine (and serotonin) at the presynaptic neuron
- May take several weeks to produce the desired effect (2 to 4 weeks after the first dose)

SCHIZOPHRENIA

- A group of mental disorders characterized by psychotic features.
  - Delusions of persecution: the client believes that he or she is being persecuted by some powerful force.
  - Delusions of grandeur: the client has an exaggerated sense of self that has no basis in reality.
  - Somatic delusions: the client believes that his or her body is changing, which has no basis in reality.
- Perceptual distortions
  - Illusions: brief experiences of misinterpretation or misperception of reality
  - Hallucinations: (five senses) with no basis in reality

Antipsychotic Medications

- Traditional medications
  - Purpose
    - Treat psychotic behavior
  - Side effects
    - Extrapyramidal
    - Anticholinergic
  - Nursing implications
    - Encourage fluid (water)
    - Gum
    - Hard candy
    - Increase fiber intake
- Long-acting medications
  - Purpose
    - Promote medication compliance
  - Side effects
    - Blood dyscrasias
    - Neuroleptic malignant syndrome
  - Nursing implications
    - Change position slowly for dizziness
    - Report urinary retention to healthcare provider
- Atypical medications
  - Purpose
    - Treat all positive and negative symptoms
  - Side effects
    - Multiple side effects depending on medication
  - Nursing implications
    - Tolerance to effects usually occurs

SUBSTANCE ABUSE DISORDERS

- Substance dependence: a pattern of repeated use of a substance.
- Substance tolerance: a need for more of the substance to reach the desired effect.
- Substance abuse: uses substance recurrently
- Substance withdrawal: symptoms occur when a drop takes place in blood levels of a substance

HESI Hint

For a client with hallucinations, safety is the first priority. Make sure that the client does not have an auditory command telling him or her to harm self or others.

HESI Hint

Neuroleptic malignant syndrome is a potentially fatal syndrome that may occur at any time during therapy with neuroleptic (antipsychotic) medications.

Alcohol Abuse

Alcohol is a central nervous system (CNS) depressant.

- Physical dependence: a biological need for alcohol to avoid physical withdrawal symptoms.
- Psychological dependence: a craving for the subjective effect of alcohol.
- Intoxication, with blood alcohol levels of 0.1% (100 mg alcohol/dL blood) or greater

ALCOHOL WITHDRAWAL

- Signs peak after 24 to 48 hours
- Chlordiazepoxide (Librium) is the most commonly prescribed medication for acute alcohol withdrawal.
- Withdrawal delirium: peaks 48 to 72 hours after cessation of intake and lasts 2 to 3 days.
  - It is a medical emergency.
  - Death can occur from myocardial infarction, fat emboli, peripheral vascular collapse, electrolyte imbalance, aspiration pneumonia, or suicide.

A male client with a history of alcohol abuse is admitted to the medical unit for GI bleeding and pancreatitis. Admission data include: BP 156/96 mm Hg, pulse 92 bpm, and temperature 99.2° F. Which is most important for the nurse to implement?
A. Provide a quiet, low-stimulus environment
B. Initiate seizure precautions
C. Administer PRN lorazepam (Ativan) as prescribed
D. Determine time and quantity of last alcohol intake

COGNITIVE IMPAIRMENT DISORDERS

Autism

- Etiology: No known cause.
- Clinical description:
  - Hyperactivity
  - Short attention span
  - Impulsivity
  - Aggressivity
  - Self-injurious behavior
  - Temper tantrums
  - Repetitive mannerisms
  - Preoccupied with objects
  - Spoken language is often absent
  - "Islands of genius."
- Prognosis: There is no cure for autism. Language skills and intellectual level are the strongest factors related to the prognosis. Only a small percentage of individuals with the disorder go on to live and work independently as adults.

Disulfiram (Antabuse) Therapy

- Alcohol deterrent
- Other medications used to assist with cravings:
  - acamprosate calcium (Campral)
  - naltrexone (ReVia)
- Instruct the client who is on disulfiram therapy to avoid the use of substances that contain alcohol, such as cough medicines, mouthwashes, and aftershave lotions.

HESI Test Question Approach		
Positive?	YES	NO
Key Words		
Rephrase		
Rule Out Choices		
A	B	C	D

118

Chapter **10** **Mental Health Nursing**

- Asperger's disorder: has many similar features of autism without significant delays in language, cognitive development, age-appropriate self-help skills, adaptive behavior, or curiosity about the environment. This disorder is lifelong.

Attention-Deficit/Hyperactivity Disorder
- Etiology: No known cause but there is a strong correlation between genetic factors and ADHD.
- Clinical description:
  — Fidgeting in a seat
  — Getting up when expected to be seated
  — Excessive running when it is dangerous or inappropriate
  — Loud and disruptive play during quiet activities
  — Forget and miss appointments
  — Fail to meet deadlines
  — Lose the train of conversation
  — Change topics inappropriately
  — Not following rules of games
- Prognosis: Continue into adolescence in the majority of children. Many adults with ADHD in childhood report a decrease of hyperactivity but a continuation of difficulty concentrating or attending to complex projects.

Dementia and Alzheimer's Disease
- Dementia is a syndrome with progressive deterioration in intellectual functioning secondary to structural or functional changes.
- Long-term and short-term memory loss
- Impairment in judgment, abstract thinking, problem-solving ability, and behavior
- The most common type of dementia is Alzheimer's disease, which is an irreversible form of senile dementia caused by nerve cell deterioration.
- Providing a safe environment is a priority in the care of a client with Alzheimer's disease.

HESI Hint
Clients with attention-deficit/hyperactivity disorder may require CNS stimulants to reduce hyperactive behavior and lengthen attention span.

Medications to Treat Alzheimer's Disease
- Donepezil (Aricept)
- Galantamine (Razadyne)
- Memantine (Namenda)
- Rivastigmine (Exelon)
- Tacrine (Cognex)

Appendix A
Normal Laboratory Values

TEST	ADULT	CHILD	INFANT/NEWBORN	ELDER	NURSING IMPLICATIONS
			HEMATOLOGICAL		
Hgb (hemo-globin): g/dL	Male: 14-18 Female: 12-16 Pregnant: >11	1-6 yr: 9.5-14 6-18 yr: 10-15.5	Newborn: 14-24 0-2 wk: 12-20 2-6 mo: 10-17 6 mo-1 yr: 9.5-14	Values slightly decreased	High-altitude living increases values. Drug therapy can alter values. Slight Hgb decreases normally occur during pregnancy.
Hct (hemat-ocrit): %	Male: 42-52 Female: 37-47 Pregnant: >33	1-6 yr: 30-40 6-18 yr: 32-44	Newborn: 44-64 2-8 wk: 39-59 2-6 mo: 35-50 6 mo-1 yr: 29-43	Values slightly decreased	Prolonged stasis from vaso-constriction secondary to the tourniquet can alter values. Abnormalities in RBC size may alter Hct values.
RBC (red blood cell) count: million/mm^3	Male: 4.7-6.1 Female: 4.2-5.4	1-6 yr: 4-5.5 6-18 yr: 4.5-5	Newborn: 4.8-7.1 2-8 wk: 4-6 2-6 mo: 3.5-5.5 6 mo-1 yr: 3.5-5.2	Same as adult	Never draw specimen from an arm with an infusing IV. Exercise and high altitudes can cause an increase in values. Pregnancy values are usually lower. Drug therapy can alter values.
WBC (white blood cell) count: 1000/mm^3	Both sexes: 5-10	≤2 yr: 6.2-17 ≥2 yr: 5-10	Newborn, term: 9-30	Same as adult	Anesthetics, stress, exercise, and convulsions can cause increased values. Drug therapy can decrease values. 24 to 48 hr postpartum; it is normal to have a count as high as 25.
Platelet count: 1000/mm^3	Both sexes: 150-400	150-400	Premature infant: 100-300 Newborn: 150-300 Infant: 200-475	Same as adult	Values may increase if living at high altitudes, exercising strenuously, or taking oral contraceptives. Values may decrease due to hemorrhage, DIC, reduced production of platelets, infections, prosthetic heart valves, and drugs (aceta-minophen, aspirin, chemo-therapy, H2 blockers, INH, Levaquin, streptomycin, sulfonamides, thiazide diuretics).

HESI Hint: Laboratory values that are most important to know for the NCLEX-PN exam are Hgb, Hct, WBCs, Na$^+$, K$^+$, BUN, blood glucose, ABGs (arterial blood gases), bilirubin for newborn, and therapeutic range for PT and PTT.

(Continued)

TEST	ADULT	CHILD	INFANT/NEWBORN	ELDER	NURSING IMPLICATIONS
SED rate, ESR (erythrocyte sedimentation rate): mm/hr	Male: up to 15 Female: up to 20 Pregnant: all trimesters	Up to 10	Newborn: 0-2	Same as adult	Rate is elevated during pregnancy.
PT (prothrombin time): sec	Both sexes: 11-12.5 Pregnant: slight ↓	Same as adult	Same as adult	Same as adult	It is used in regulating Coumadin therapy. Therapeutic range is 1.5 to 2 times normal or control.
PTT (partial thromboplastin time): sec (see APTT)	Both sexes: 60-70 Pregnant: slight ↓	Same as adult	Same as adult	Same as adult	It is used in regulating heparin therapy. Therapeutic range is 1.5 to 2.5 times normal or control.
APTT (activated partial thromboplastin time): sec	Both sexes: 30-40	Same as adult	Same as adult	Same as adult	It is used in regulating heparin therapy. Therapeutic range is 1.5 to 2.5 times normal or control.
BLOOD CHEMISTRY					
Alkaline phosphatase: IU/L	Both sexes: 30-120	2-8 yr: 65-210 9-15 yr: 60-300 16-21 yr: 30-200	<2 yr: 85-235	Slightly higher than adult	Hemolysis of specimen can cause a false elevation in values.
Albumin: g/dL	Both sexes: 3.5-5 Pregnant: slight	4.5-9	Premature infant: 3-4.2 Newborn: 3.5-5.4 Infant: 6-6.7	Same as adult	No special preparation is needed.
Bilirubin total: mg/dL	Total: 0.3-1 Indirect: 0.2-0.8 Direct: 0.1-0.3	Same as adult	Newborn: 1-12	Same as adult	Client is to be NPO except for water for 8 to 12 hr before testing. Prevent hemolysis of blood during venipuncture. Do *not* shake tube; it can cause inaccurate values. Protect blood sample from bright light.
Calcium: mg/dL	Both sexes: 9-10.5	8.8-10.8	<10 days: 7.6-10.4 Umbilical: 9-11.5 10 days-2 yr: 9-10.6	Values tend to decrease	No special preparation is needed. Use of thiazide diuretics can cause increased calcium values.
Chloride: mEq/L	Both sexes: 98-106	90-110	Newborn: 96-106 Premature infant: 95-110	Same as adult	Do not collect from an arm with an infusing IV solution.
Cholesterol: mg/dL	Both sexes: <200	120-200	Infant: 70-175 Newborn: 53-135	Same as adult	Do not collect from an arm with an infusing IV solution.

(Continued)

TEST	ADULT	CHILD	INFANT/NEWBORN	ELDER	NURSING IMPLICATIONS
CPK (creatine phosphoki-nase): IU/L	Male: 55-170 Female: 30-135	Same as adult	Newborn: 65-580	Same as adult	Specimen must not be stored before running test.
Creatinine: mg/dL	Male: 0.6-1.2 Female: 0.5-1.1	Child: 0.3-0.7 Adolescent: 0.5-1	Newborn: 0.2-0.4 Infant: 0.3-1.2	Decrease in muscle mass may cause decreased values	It is preferred but not neces-sary to be NPO 8 hr before testing. A ratio of 20:1 BUN to cre-atinine indicates adequate kidney functioning.
Glucose: mg/dL	Both sexes: 70-110	≤2 yr: 60-100 >2 yr: 7	Cord: 45-96 Premature infant: 20-60 Newborn: 30-60 Infant: 40-90	Increase in normal range after age 50	Client to be NPO except for water 8 hr before testing. Caffeine can cause increased values.
HCO_3^-: mEq/L	Both sexes: 23-30	20-28	Newborn: 13-22 Infant: 20-28	Same as adult	None
Iron: µg/dL	Male: 80-180 Female: 60-160	50-120	Newborn: 100-250	Same as adult	It is preferred but not neces-sary to be NPO 8 hr before testing.
TIBC (total iron binding capac-ity): µg/dL	Both sexes: 250-460	Same as adult	Same as adult	Same as adult	None
LDH (lactic dehydroge-nase): IU/L	Both sexes: 100-190	60-170	Newborn: 160-450 Infant: 100-250	Same as adult	No IM injections are to be given 8 to 12 hr before test-ing. Hemolysis of blood will cause false positive result.
Potassium: mEq/L	Both sexes: 3.5-5	3.4-4.7	Newborn: 3-5.9 Infant: 4.1-5.3	Same as adult	Hemolysis of specimen can result in falsely elevated values. Exercise of the forearm with tourniquet in place may cause an increased potas-sium level.
Protein total: g/dL	Both sexes: 6.4-8.3	6.2-8	Premature infant: 4.2-7.6 Newborn: 4.6-7.4 Infant: 6-6.7	Same as adult	It is preferred but not neces-sary to be NPO 8 hr before testing.
AST/SGOT (aspartate ami-notransferase): IU/L	0-35 Female slightly lower than adult males	3-6 yr: 15-50 6-12 yr: 10-50 12-18 yr: 10-40	0-5 days: 35-140 <3 yr: 15-60	Slightly higher than adult	Hemolysis of specimen can result in falsely elevated values. Exercise may cause an increased value.
ALT/SGPT (alanine ami-notransferase): IU/mL	Both sexes: 4-36	Same as adult	Infant may be twice as high as adult	Slightly higher than adult	Hemolysis of specimen can result in falsely elevated values. Exercise may cause an increased value

(Continued)

Appendix **A** **Normal Laboratory Values**

TEST	ADULT	CHILD	INFANT/NEWBORN	ELDER	NURSING IMPLICATIONS
Sodium: mEq/L	Both sexes: 136-145	136-145	Newborn: 134-144 Infant: 134-150	Same as adult	Do not collect from an arm with an infusing IV solution.
Triglycerides: mg/dL	Male: 40-160 Female: 35-135	6-11 yr: 31-108 12-15 yr: 36-138 16-19 yr: 40-163	0-5 yr: 30-86	Same as adult	Client is to be NPO 12 hr before testing. No alcohol for 24 hr before test.
BUN (blood urea nitrogen): mg/dL	Both sexes: 10-20	5-18	Newborn: 3-12 Cord: 21-40 Infant: 5-18	Slightly higher	None
ARTERIAL BLOOD CHEMISTRY					
pH	Both sexes: 7.35-7.45	Same as adult	Newborn: 3-12 Cord: 21-40 Infant: 5-18	Same as adult	Specimen must be heparinized. Specimen must be iced for transport. All air bubbles must be expelled from sample. Direct pressure to puncture site must be maintained.
Pco_2: mm Hg	Both sexes: 35-45	Same as adult	<2 yr: 26-41	Same as adult	Specimen must be heparinized. Specimen must be iced for transport. All air bubbles must be expelled from sample. Direct pressure to puncture site must be maintained.
Po_2: mm Hg	Both sexes: 80-100	Same as adult	Newborn: 60-70	Same as adult	Specimen must be heparinized. Specimen must be iced for transport. All air bubbles must be expelled from sample. Direct pressure to puncture site must be maintained.
Hco_3^-: mEq/L	Both sexes: 21-28	Same as adult	Infant/newborn: 16-24	Same as adult	Specimen must be heparinized. Specimen must be iced for transport. All air bubbles must be expelled from sample. Direct pressure to puncture site must be maintained.
O_2 Saturation: %	Both sexes: 95-100	Same as adult	Newborn: 40-90	95	Specimen must be heparinized. Specimen must be iced for transport. All air bubbles must be expelled from sample. Direct pressure to puncture site must be maintained.

From Pagana, T.J., & Pagana, K.D. (2007). *Mosby's diagnostic and laboratory test reference* (8th ed.). St Louis: Mosby.

NCLEX-RN® Examination Practice Questions

Management/Leadership

1. **Which activity should the nurse delegate to an unlicensed assistive personnel (UAP)?**
   A. Check a client with cirrhosis to see if he can hear any better today after an IV antibiotic was discontinued.
   B. Push additional PO fluids for an elderly client with pneumonia who has developed a fever.
   C. Report the ability of a client with myasthenia gravis to manage the supper tray independently.
   D. Measure the liquid stool of a client who has received lactulose for an elevated serum NH3 level.

HESI Test Question Approach		
Positive?	YES	NO
Key Words		
Rephrase		
Rule Out Choices		
A	B	C	D

2. **The nurse is delegating several client problems to the UAP. Which client requires the nurse to intervene? The client with**
   A. Active TB who is leaving the room without a mask.
   B. Dehydration who is requesting something to drink.
   C. Asthma who complains of being anxious and cannot concentrate.
   D. COPD who is leaving the unit to smoke as the next IVPB is due.

HESI Test Question Approach		
Positive?	YES	NO
Key Words		
Rephrase		
Rule Out Choices		
A	B	C	D

3. **The nurse reports that a female client plans to unscrew the light bulb in her room and try to cut herself. How should the charge nurse plan for nursing care?**
   A. Call in an extra nurse or technician for the next shift.
   B. Assign one of the current staff to be with the client.
   C. Move the client to another room with a roommate.
   D. The charge nurse should plan to care for this client.

HESI Test Question Approach		
Positive?	YES	NO
Key Words		
Rephrase		
Rule Out Choices		
A	B	C	D

4. The UAP is assisting with the care of eight clients on a postpartum unit. Which assignment should the nurse delegate to the UAP?

A. Check fundal firmness and lochia for the clients who delivered vaginally.

B. Take vital signs q 15 min for a client with preeclampsia.

C. Provide breast-feeding instructions for a primigravida.

D. Assist with daily care activities for clients on bed rest.

HESI Test Question Approach			
Positive?		YES	NO
Key Words			
Rephrase			
Rule Out Choices			
A	B	C	D

Advanced Clinical Concepts

5. Which client is at the highest risk for respiratory complications?

A. An 18-year-old with dehydration and cerebral palsy who is dependent in daily activities.

B. A 60-year-old client with IDDM for 20 years who is admitted with cellulitis of the left leg.

C. An obese 30-year-old with hypertension who is noncompliant with the medication regimen.

D. A 40-year-old with a serum K^+ of 3.4 mEq/L who complains of fatigue while taking a loop diuretic.

HESI Test Question Approach			
Positive?		YES	NO
Key Words			
Rephrase			
Rule Out Choices			
A	B	C	D

6. A nurse stops at an accident and finds a young adult male in an overturned truck that is leaking gasoline onto the hot pavement. The victim is pulseless and apneic. What action has the highest priority?

A. Initiate basic life support.

B. Remove the victim from the truck.

C. Assess for hemorrhage.

D. Remove glass shards from the face.

HESI Test Question Approach			
Positive?		YES	NO
Key Words			
Rephrase			
Rule Out Choices			
A	B	C	D

7. The nurse observes that the IV infusion is empty for a client who has been vomiting during the immediate postoperative period. What action should the nurse implement?
A. Hang a liter of D_5 ½ NS at the current rate.
B. Use normal saline (NS) or lock the IV access.
C. Maintain the infusion using a liter of ½ NS.
D. Start a liter of D_5 LR at a keep-open rate.

HESI Test Question Approach		
Positive?	YES	NO
Key Words		
Rephrase		
Rule Out Choices		
A	B	C	D

8. The nurse is administering a prescription for clotting factors for a client in shock. For which problem should the nurse plan the focus of care?
A. Cardiac output
B. Fluid volume deficit
C. Infection
D. Peripheral perfusion

HESI Test Question Approach		
Positive?	YES	NO
Key Words		
Rephrase		
Rule Out Choices		
A	B	C	D

9. A client's arterial blood gas results are pH 7.29, Pco_2 55 mm Hg, and Hco_3- 26 mEq/L. Which compensatory response should the nurse expect this client to exhibit?
A. Tachypnea
B. Tachycardia
C. Increased blood pressure
D. Cerebral vasodilation

HESI Test Question Approach		
Positive?	YES	NO
Key Words		
Rephrase		
Rule Out Choices		
A	B	C	D

10. **A client who has chronic back pain is not receiving adequate pain relief from oral analgesics. What alternative action should the nurse explore to promote the client's comfort and independence?**
   A. Ask the healthcare provider to increase the analgesic dosage.
   B. Secure a prescription for a second analgesic by IV route.
   C. Consider the client's receptivity to using a TENS unit.
   D. Encourage counseling to avoid future addiction.

HESI Test Question Approach		
Positive?		YES NO
Key Words		
Rephrase		
Rule Out Choices		
A	B	C D

Maternal/Newborn Nursing

11. **A 40-week gestational client is in active labor and calls the nurse to report her membranes ruptured. The nurse performs a sterile vaginal examination and discovers a prolapsed umbilical cord. Which intervention should the nurse implement first?**
   A. Elevate the presenting fetal part off the cord.
   B. Cover the cord with sterile warm NS gauze.
   C. Prepare for an emergency cesarean birth.
   D. Start O_2 by facemask at 10 L/min.

HESI Test Question Approach		
Positive?		YES NO
Key Words		
Rephrase		
Rule Out Choices		
A	B	C D

12. **A 39-week gestational client plans to have an epidural block when labor is established. What intervention should the nurse implement to prevent side effects?**
   A. Teach about the procedure and effects of the epidural.
   B. Maintain the epidural infusion continuously throughout the second stage of labor.
   C. Administer a bolus of 500 to 1000 mL of a non-dextrose saline solution.
   D. Take vital signs every 30 minutes after the epidural medication is injected.

HESI Test Question Approach		
Positive?		YES NO
Key Words		
Rephrase		
Rule Out Choices		
A	B	C D

NCLEX-RN® Examination Practice Questions

13. A female client presents in the emergency department complaining of RLQ abdominal pain and pain in her right shoulder. She has no vaginal bleeding, and her last menses was 6 weeks ago. Which action should the nurse implement first?
    A. Assess for abdominal rebound pain, distention, and fever.
    B. Obtain VS, IV access, and notify the healthcare provider.
    C. Observe for recent musculoskeletal injury, bruising, or abuse.
    D. Collect specimens for pregnancy test, hemoglobin, and WBC count.

HESI Test Question Approach			
Positive?		YES	NO
Key Words			
Rephrase			
Rule Out Choices			
A	B	C	D

14. A pregnant client with class III cardiac disease has hemoglobin of 10g and a hematocrit of 28.7%. The nurse instructs the client to double her iron supplement, and she complains the extra iron will make her constipated. What explanation should the nurse offer?
    A. Constipation is caused by rising pregnancy hormones and crowding of the growing fetus, not the iron.
    B. Labor increases the workload of the heart, so stop the supplements 1 week before your due date.
    C. Anemia stresses the heart to work harder, so an abundant iron intake is needed to synthesize red blood cells.
    D. Bleeding during labor and delivery is expected and additional iron will be needed for erythropoiesis.

HESI Test Question Approach			
Positive?		YES	NO
Key Words			
Rephrase			
Rule Out Choices			
A	B	C	D

Medical/Surgical Renal

15. A client is returning to the unit after an intravenous pyelogram (IVP). Which intervention should the nurse include in the plan of care?
    A. Maintain bed rest
    B. Increase fluid intake
    C. Monitor for hematuria
    D. Continue NPO status

HESI Test Question Approach			
Positive?		YES	NO
Key Words			
Rephrase			
Rule Out Choices			
A	B	C	D

16. The nurse is teaching a client who has chronic urinary tract infections about a prescription for ciprofloxacin (Cipro) 500 mg PO bid. What side effect should the client not expect during the duration of medication therapy?
A. Photosensitivity
B. Dyspepsia
C. Diarrhea
D. Urinary frequency

HESI Test Question Approach			
Positive?		YES	NO
Key Words			
Rephrase			
Rule Out Choices			
A	B	C	D

17. Which client's complaints of pain require the nurse's intervention first? A client who is complaining of
A. Bladder pain while receiving a continuous saline irrigant 2 hours after a transurethral prostatic resection.
B. Incisional pain on the third day postnephrectomy and requesting a PRN oral pain medication.
C. Flank pain that is partially relieved after passing a renal calculus.
D. Bladder spasms after draining 1000 mL of urine during insertion of an indwelling catheter.

HESI Test Question Approach			
Positive?		YES	NO
Key Words			
Rephrase			
Rule Out Choices			
A	B	C	D

18. A male client with a Tenckhoff catheter calls to report he feels "poorly" and has a fever. What is the best response by the clinic nurse?
A. Encourage him to come to the clinic today for assessment.
B. Instruct him to increase his fluid intake to 3 L/day.
C. Review his medication regimen for compliance.
D. Inquire about his recent dietary intake of protein and iron.

HESI Test Question Approach			
Positive?		YES	NO
Key Words			
Rephrase			
Rule Out Choices			
A	B	C	D

Medical/Surgical Cardiovascular

19. The nurse is reviewing the cardiac markers for a client who is admitted after reporting chest pain that occurred last week. Which laboratory value elevation should the nurse identify as a late marker after myocardial injury?
    A. Troponin level
    B. Myoglobin level
    C. CK-MB levels
    D. LDH levels

HESI Test Question Approach			
Positive?		YES	NO
Key Words			
Rephrase			
Rule Out Choices			
A	B	C	D

20. The nurse is providing discharge instructions to a client who is diagnosed with angina pectoris. Which instruction is most important?
    A. Avoid activity that will involve the Valsalva maneuver.
    B. Seek emergency treatment if chest pain persists after the third nitroglycerin dose.
    C. Rest for 30 minutes after having chest pain before resuming activity.
    D. Keep extra nitroglycerin in an airtight and light-resistant bottle.

HESI Test Question Approach			
Positive?		YES	NO
Key Words			
Rephrase			
Rule Out Choices			
A	B	C	D

21. The nurse is providing discharge teaching for a client who is prescribed diltiazem (Cardizem). Which dietary instruction has the highest priority?
    A. Maintain a low-sodium diet
    B. Eat a banana each morning
    C. Ingest high-fiber foods daily
    D. Avoid grapefruit products

HESI Test Question Approach			
Positive?		YES	NO
Key Words			
Rephrase			
Rule Out Choices			
A	B	C	D

22. **The nurse is teaching a young adult female who has a history of Raynaud's disease how to control her pain. What information should the nurse offer?**
   A. Take oral analgesic at regularly spaced intervals.
   B. Avoid extremes of heat and cold.
   C. Limit foods and fluids with caffeine.
   D. Keep involved extremities in a dependent position.

HESI Test Question Approach		
Positive?	YES	NO
Key Words		
Rephrase		
Rule Out Choices		
A	B	C	D

23. **The nurse is planning care for a client who is admitted with thrombocytopenia. Which nursing diagnosis best addresses this client's problem?**
   A. Infection, risk for
   B. Injury, risk for bleeding
   C. Impaired nutrition, less than requirements
   D. Fatigue

HESI Test Question Approach		
Positive?	YES	NO
Key Words		
Rephrase		
Rule Out Choices		
A	B	C	D

Medical/Surgical Respiratory

24. **A client who is admitted with cancer of the larynx is scheduled for a laryngectomy tomorrow. What is the top learning need for the client tonight?**
   A. Body image counseling
   B. Pain management expectations
   C. Communication techniques
   D. Postoperative nutritional needs

HESI Test Question Approach		
Positive?	YES	NO
Key Words		
Rephrase		
Rule Out Choices		
A	B	C	D

Psychiatric Nursing

25. A victim of a motor vehicle collision arrives in the emergency department dead on arrival. What action should the nurse implement to assist the spouse with this crisis?

A. Ask if there are family, friends, or clergy to call.

B. Talk about the former relationship with the spouse.

C. Provide education about the stages of grief and loss.

D. Assess the spouse's level of anxiety.

HESI Test Question Approach		
Positive?	YES	NO
Key Words		
Rephrase		
Rule Out Choices		
A	B	C	D

26. The nurse is planning to lead a seminar for clinic and community health nurses on violence against women during pregnancy. Which statement describes an appropriate technique to assess for violence?

A. Women should be assessed only if they are part of a high-risk group.

B. Women may be assessed in the presence of young children, but not intimate partners.

C. Women should be assessed once during pregnancy.

D. Women should be reassessed face to face by a nurse as the pregnancy progresses.

HESI Test Question Approach		
Positive?	YES	NO
Key Words		
Rephrase		
Rule Out Choices		
A	B	C	D

27. The charge nurse reminds several clients on the mental health unit that breakfast is at 8 AM, medications are given at 9 AM, and group therapy sessions begin at 10 AM. Which treatment modality has been implemented?

A. Milieu therapy

B. Behavior modification

C. Peer therapy

D. Problem solving

HESI Test Question Approach		
Positive?	YES	NO
Key Words		
Rephrase		
Rule Out Choices		
A	B	C	D

28. The nurse is accompanying a male client to x-ray when he becomes panic stricken at the elevator and states, "I can't get on that elevator." Which action should the nurse implement first?
   A. Ask one more staff member to ride in the elevator.
   B. Offer an antianxiety medication.
   C. Begin desensitization about riding the elevator.
   D. Affirm his fears about riding the elevator.

HESI Test Question Approach			
Positive?		YES	NO
Key Words			
Rephrase			
Rule Out Choices			
A	B	C	D

29. A male client who experiences frequent nightmares and somnambulism is found one night trying to strangle his roommate. Which action that the nurse should implement has the highest priority?
   A. Give the client a sedative.
   B. Administer an antipsychotic.
   C. Move the client to a different room.
   D. Process with both clients about the event.

HESI Test Question Approach			
Positive?		YES	NO
Key Words			
Rephrase			
Rule Out Choices			
A	B	C	D

30. The nurse is updating the plan of care for a client who has a borderline personality disorder. Which intervention should be included with the nursing diagnosis of ineffective coping related to manipulation?
   A. Refer the client's requests to one nurse.
   B. Avoid challenging inappropriate behavior.
   C. Limit client's contact with other clients.
   D. Remove consequences for acting-out behaviors.

HESI Test Question Approach			
Positive?		YES	NO
Key Words			
Rephrase			
Rule Out Choices			
A	B	C	D

31. **A female adolescent is admitted to the mental health unit for anorexia nervosa. What is the nurse's priority intervention?**
A. Teach about the importance of self-expression.
B. Supervise activities during the day.
C. Include in daily group therapy.
D. Facilitate social interactions with others.

HESI Test Question Approach			
Positive?		YES	NO
Key Words			
Rephrase			
Rule Out Choices			
A	B	C	D

32. **The charge nurse is planning the daily schedule for clients on the mental health unit. To which activity group should a male client who is manic be assigned?**
A. Basketball game in the gym.
B. Jogging at least 1 mile.
C. Ping-pong game with peer.
D. Group therapy with the art therapist.

HESI Test Question Approach			
Positive?		YES	NO
Key Words			
Rephrase			
Rule Out Choices			
A	B	C	D

ANSWERS AND RATIONALES

(Correct answers are underlined)

Management/Leadership

1. Which activity should the nurse delegate to an unlicensed assistive personnel (UAP)?

Rationales:

A. *Check a client with cirrhosis to see if he can hear any better today after an IV antibiotic was discontinued.*
This requires assessment about ototoxicity, which is beyond the scope of the UAP.

B. *Push additional PO fluids for an elderly client with pneumonia who has developed a fever.*
These directions are not sufficiently clear and detailed for the UAP to perform the task.

C. *Report the ability of a client with myasthenia gravis to manage the supper tray independently.*
This requires assessment of the client's clinical status that is beyond the scope of the UAP.

D. <u>*Measure the liquid stool of a client who has received lactulose for an increased serum NH3 level.*</u>
This task encompasses basic care, elimination, and intake and output; it does not require judgment or the expertise of the nurse and can be performed by the UAP.

2. The nurse is delegating several client problems to the UAP. Which client requires the nurse to intervene? The client with

Rationales:

A. *Active TB who is leaving the room without a mask.*
A UAP can be delegated to provide a box of masks, or to direct the client back to the room.

B. *Dehydration who is requesting something to drink.*
A UAP can be directed to provide specific types and amounts of fluids.

C. <u>*Asthma who complains of being anxious and cannot concentrate.*</u>
This client requires assessment and is at risk for airway compromise, which also requires assessment, so the nurse should respond to this client first.

D. *COPD who is leaving the unit to smoke as the next IVPB is due.*
A UAP can ask the client to delay leaving the unit.

3. The nurse reports that a female client plans to unscrew the light bulb in her room and try to cut herself. How should the charge nurse plan for nursing care?

Rationales:

A. *Call in an extra nurse or technician for the next shift.*
The charge nurse should plan ahead for staffing, but the immediate focus should be the client's safety now.

B. <u>*Assign one of the current staff to be with the client.*</u>
Since the client is at risk for suicide, the charge nurse should assign a staff member to stay with the client.

C. *Move the client to another room with a roommate.*
This will not ensure the client's safety, and a staff member must be present with the client at all times, not another client.

D. *The charge nurse should plan to care for this client.*
The charge nurse should not assume responsibility for the care of an individual client, since additional management responsibilities may interfere with the ability to ensure safe care.

4. The UAP is assisting with the care of eight clients on a postpartum unit. Which assignment should the nurse delegate to the UAP?

Rationales:

A. *Check fundal firmness and lochia for the clients who delivered vaginally.*
Assessment is a responsibility of the nurse.

B. *Take vital signs every 15 minutes for a client with preeclampsia.*
This is a high-risk patient who needs to be evaluated by a licensed nurse.

C. *Provide breast-feeding instructions for a primigravida.*
Teaching is also the responsibility of the RN.

D. <u>*Assist with daily care activities for clients on bed rest.*</u>
This is the most appropriate assignment for the UAP. The RN should delegate daily care activities to the UAP based on the RN's assessments of each client's needs.

Advanced Clinical Concepts

5. Which client is at the highest risk for respiratory complications?

Rationales:

A. <u>*An 18-year-old with dehydration and cerebral palsy who is dependent in daily activities.*</u>
A client with dehydration and cerebral palsy (characterized by uncoordinated and spastic muscle movements) that causes significant involvement to affect ADL independence is at an increased risk for respiratory problems due to impaired mobility and impaired swallowing.

B. *A 60-year-old with IDDM for 20 years who is admitted with cellulitis of the left leg.*
This older client is more at risk for renal, cardiac, and vascular complications.

C. *An obese 30-year-old with hypertension who is noncompliant with the medication regimen.*
An obese adult who is noncompliant with antihypertensive medications is more at risk for cardiac or cerebral events than for respiratory problems.

D. *A 40-year-old with a serum K^+ of 3.4mEq/L who complains of fatigue while taking a loop diuretic.*
This middle-aged adult is hypokalemic and fatigued, but is not at high risk for respiratory problems.

6. **A nurse stops at an accident and finds a young adult male in an overturned truck that is leaking gasoline onto the hot pavement. The victim is pulseless and apneic. What action has the highest priority?**

Rationales:
A. *Initiate basic life support.*
Although initiating CPR is vital to this victim's survival, it is not the first priority when there is the risk of explosion and fire.
B. *Remove the victim from the truck.*
The top priority is to remove the victim from the unsafe situation.
C. *Assess for hemorrhage.*
Accident victims are at risk for internal or external hemorrhage; however, this assessment does not have the highest priority.
D. *Remove glass shards from the face.*
Other life-threatening situations require action before the removal of glass.

7. **The nurse observes that the IV infusion is empty for a client who has been vomiting during the immediate postoperative period. What action should the nurse implement?**

Rationales:
A. *Hang a liter of D$_5$ ½ NS at the current rate.*
This action is not recommended because hypertonic solutions are prescribed for fluid and electrolyte imbalances and cause an osmotic movement of fluids into the vasculature.
B. *Use normal saline (NS) or lock the IV access.*
The nurse should maintain the IV access with an isotonic solution, such as NS, for intravascular fluid volume replacement or lock the access until further prescriptions are available.
C. *Maintain the infusion with a liter of ½ NS.*
This is not a recommended action because this hypotonic solution is prescribed for cellular dehydration, not postoperative fluid volume deficit.
D. *Start a liter of D$_5$ LR at a keep-open rate.*
This is not a recommended action because a hypertonic solution will cause an osmotic movement of fluids into the vascular space and contribute to fluid and electrolyte imbalances.

8. **The nurse is administering a prescription for clotting factors for a client in shock. For which problem should the nurse plan the focus of care?**

Rationales:
A. *Cardiac output*
Cardiogenic shock is the result of the heart failing as a pump.
B. *Fluid volume deficit*
Hypovolemic shock is the result of fluid volume loss, either from the body or due to third spacing.
C. *Infection*
The nurse should focus the plan of care on infection. Septic shock results from toxins circulating in the

vascular bed that cause the clotting factors to pool in the microcirculation, leaving the client vulnerable to bleeding due to insufficient factors in the larger vessels, i.e., disseminating intravascular coagulation (DIC).
D. *Peripheral perfusion*
Vasogenic shock is similar to hypovolemic shock because generalized vasodilation results in insufficient blood volume in the "now" enlarged vascular tree, which results in a reduced hydrostatic pressure with inadequate baroreceptor response.

9. **A client's arterial blood gas results are pH 7.29, Pco$_2$ 55 mm Hg, and Hco$_3^-$ 26 mEq/L. Which compensatory response should the nurse expect this client to exhibit?**

Rationales:
A. *Tachypnea*
The client is experiencing respiratory acidosis and will demonstrate hyperventilation as a compensatory mechanism to remove excess CO$_2$.
B. *Tachycardia*
Acid-base imbalances are compensated primarily by the lungs and the renal system. Plasma proteins and ionic shifts (intracellular) also serve as buffering systems. Tachycardia (B), increased BP (C), and cerebral vasodilation (D) do not serve as compensatory mechanisms.
C. *Increased blood pressure*
See rationale for option B.
D. *Cerebral vasodilation*
See rationale for option B.

10. **A client who has chronic back pain is not receiving adequate pain relief from oral analgesics. What alternative action should the nurse explore to promote the client's comfort and independence?**

Rationales:
A. *Ask the healthcare provider to increase the analgesic dosage.*
While this intervention may improve pain relief, it may not promote self-care without increasing side effects that may affect the client's independence.
B. *Secure a prescription for a second analgesic by IV route.*
The IV route does not promote self-care and also may cause additional side effects that interfere with the client's ability to carry out ADLs independently.
C. *Consider the client's receptivity to use a TENS unit.*
This action supports increased pain control and self-care without the high level of adverse effects associated with additional medication. It is the least invasive measure, and promotes the active participation (self-care) of the client.
D. *Encourage counseling to avoid future addiction.*
Referrals may be needed, but the nurse should teach clients about potential problems with medications and measures to manage pain and maintain self-care.

Maternal/Newborn Nursing

11. A 40-week gestational client is in active labor and calls the nurse to report her membrane has ruptured. The nurse performs a sterile vaginal examination and discovers a prolapsed umbilical cord. Which intervention should the nurse implement first?

Rationales:

A. *Elevate the presenting fetal part off the cord.*
This action is the most critical intervention; the nurse must prevent compression of the cord by the presenting part, which will impair fetal circulation, leading to both morbidity and death.

B. *Cover the cord with sterile warm NS gauze.*
If the cord is protruding outside the vagina, this should be implemented to prevent drying of the Wharton's jelly. However, another nurse should do this while the nurse maintains elevation of the presenting part off the cord.

C. *Prepare for an emergency cesarean birth.*
This is implemented by the staff while the nurse maintains the presenting part off the cord.

D. *Start O₂ by facemask at 10 L/min.*
Oxygen should be provided to the mother to increase oxygen delivery to the fetus via the placenta, but another nurse should implement this while the nurse maintains the presenting part off the cord.

12. A 39-week gestational client plans to have an epidural block when labor is established. What intervention should the nurse implement to prevent side effects?

Rationales:

A. *Teach about the procedure and effects of the epidural.*
Teaching is an important nursing intervention to alleviate anxiety, but it does not prevent hypotension, a side effect due to vasodilation caused by the epidural block.

B. *Maintain the epidural infusion continuously throughout the second stage of labor.*
Difficulty in internal rotation of the fetal head may occur because of relaxation of the pelvic floor, caused by the epidural, and therefore it may be necessary to discontinue the epidural infusion during transition or at the end of stage I.

C. *Administer a bolus of 500 to 1000 mL of a nondextrose saline solution.*
Prehydration will increase maternal blood volume and prevent hypotension, which occurs due to vasodilation, a side effect of epidural anesthesia. A nondextrose solution is used to prevent fetal secretion of insulin that later places the neonate at risk for hypoglycemia.

D. *Take vital signs every 30 minutes after the epidural medication is injected.*
Vital signs should be monitored every 5 minutes immediately after the initial epidural dose, and if stable, then every 15 minutes.

13. A female client presents in the emergency department complaining of RLQ abdominal pain and pain in her right shoulder. She has no vaginal bleeding, and her last menses was 6 weeks ago. Which action should the nurse implement first?

Rationales:

A. *Assess for abdominal rebound pain, distention, and fever.*
Bleeding related to an ectopic pregnancy (based on the client's history) may present these manifestations, but the nurse should first assess the client for hypovolemic shock.

B. *Obtain VS, IV access, and notify the healthcare provider.*
The nurse should first evaluate the client for vital sign changes of shock due to a ruptured ectopic pregnancy (an obstetrical emergency). A vascular access is vital in an emergency situation, and the healthcare provider should be notified immediately.

C. *Observe for recent musculoskeletal injury, bruising, or abuse.*
This may be part of the assessment if a life-threatening situation is ruled out first.

D. *Collect specimens for pregnancy test, hemoglobin, and WBC count.*
A pregnancy test and CBC specimens should be collected, but the nurse should first notify the healthcare provider of the client's status based on the presenting vital signs and symptoms of bleeding, as manifested by intraabdominal bleeding that collects under the diaphragm causing referred shoulder pain.

14. A pregnant client with class III cardiac disease has a hemoglobin of 10 g and a hematocrit of 28.7%. The nurse instructs the client to double her iron supplement; she complains the extra iron will make her constipated. What explanation should the nurse offer?

Rationales:

A. *Constipation is caused by rising pregnancy hormones and crowding of the growing fetus, not the iron.*
Oral iron supplements cause the stool to become tenacious and contribute to constipation.

B. *Labor increases the workload of the heart, so stop the supplements 1 week before your due date.*
This does not explain the need for the additional iron.

C. *Anemia stresses the heart to work harder, so extra iron is needed to synthesize red blood cells.*
The nurse should explain that the heart works harder to pump inadequate numbers of RBCs, so extra iron is needed to produce more cells to carry adequate oxygen to tissues and thereby reduce the workload of the heart.

D. *Bleeding during labor and delivery is expected and additional iron will be needed for erythropoiesis.*
Additional iron should be made available for erythropoiesis, after delivery; however, the client's cardiac disease is the underlying reason to treat anemia.

Medical/Surgical Renal

15. A client is returning to the unit after an intravenous pyelogram (IVP). Which intervention should the nurse include in the plan of care?

Rationales:

A. *Maintain bed rest*
There is no need to restrict mobility after an IVP.

B. *Increase fluid intake*
The client should increase the intake of fluids to adequately clear the dye used in an IVP because the dye may damage the kidneys.

C. *Monitor for hematuria*
There is no risk of hematuria related to the IVP.

D. *Continue NPO status*
The client does not need to be NPO after an IVP. Fluids should be increased.

16. The nurse is teaching a client who has chronic urinary tract infections about a prescription for ciprofloxacin (Cipro) 500 mg PO bid. What side effect should the client not expect during the duration of medication therapy?

Rationales:

A. *Photosensitivity*
This is a side effect of Cipro and the nurse should instruct clients to avoid exposure to the sun.

B. *Dyspepsia*
Cipro causes GI irritation, nausea and vomiting, and abdominal pain, which should be reported.

C. *Diarrhea*
Watery, foul-smelling diarrhea is an adverse reaction of Cipro that is an indicator of pseudomembranous colitis, which should be reported and requires immediate intervention.

D. *Urinary frequency*
Urinary frequency is not a side effect of Cipro yet this symptom may indicate that the medication is ineffective and should be reported.

17. Which client's complaints of pain require the nurse's intervention first? A client who is complaining of

Rationales:

A. *Bladder pain while receiving a continuous saline irrigant 2 hours after a transurethral prostatic resection.*
This client is at risk of clot formation occluding the catheter, which may indicate bleeding and bladder distention, and the nurse should evaluate this client immediately.

B. *Incisional pain on the third day after a nephrectomy and requesting a PRN oral pain medication.*
This is not as high a priority compared to option A because the client is not at risk of any altered homeostasis.

C. *Flank pain that is partially relieved after passing a renal calculus.*
This client's condition is not likely to worsen now that the stone was passed, and should be evaluated after the client in option A.

D. *Bladder spasms after draining 1000 mL of urine during insertion of an indwelling catheter.*
This client's pain reflects bladder spasms and is of lower priority than option A.

18. A male client with a Tenckhoff catheter calls to report he feels "poorly" and has a fever. What is the best response by the clinic nurse?

Rationales:

A. *Encourage him to come to the clinic today for assessment.*
Tenckhoff catheters are used in peritoneal dialysis. They are often used at home by the client, placing the client at risk for peritoneal infection. Because dialysis clients usually have some degree of compromised immunity and anemia, he should be assessed and should come to the clinic.

B. *Instruct him to increase his fluid intake to 3 L/day.*
Clients who need dialysis retain fluid and usually are restricted to a 300-mL intake greater than output.

C. *Review his medication regimen for compliance.*
The nurse should evaluate the client's compliance, but assessing the client for infection is a greater priority.

D. *Inquire about his recent dietary intake of protein and iron.*
Iron deficiency and protein loss are common problems in clients who are receiving peritoneal dialysis. Dietary intake is important but does not hold a higher priority than possible infection.

Medical/Surgical Cardiovascular

19. The nurse is reviewing the cardiac markers for a client who is admitted after reporting chest pain that occurred last week. Which laboratory value elevation should the nurse identify as a late marker after myocardial injury?

Rationales:

A. *Troponin level*
Troponin is released quickly from the injured myocardial tissue but will fall after 5-14 days and slowly return to normal levels; Troponin levels are the most immediate and specific cardiac biomarkers but are useful as a delayed indicator of myocardial injury.

B. *Myoglobin level*
Whole myoglobin starts to increase in about 3 hours after MI, but it is not as sensitive as other markers and can rise even after skeletal muscle injury, such as occurs with IM injection, and returns to normal in 2 days.

C. *CK-MB levels*
This isoenzyme is useful in supporting MI, determining the extent and time of the infarct. This marker usually returns to normal in 72 hours and is less useful in the nonacute phase.

D. *LDH levels*
Elevated LDH levels are risk factors for cardiovascular lesions.

139

20. The nurse is providing discharge instructions to a client who is diagnosed with angina pectoris. Which instruction is most important?

Rationales:

A. *Avoid activity that will involve the Valsalva maneuver.*
While minimizing or avoiding the Valsalva maneuver will decrease anginal pain, it is not the most important factor.

B. *Seek emergency treatment if chest pain persists after the third nitroglycerin dose.*
This instruction has the most importance because chest pain characteristic of acute MI persists longer than 15 minutes, and delaying medical treatment can be life threatening.

C. *Rest for 30 minutes after having chest pain before resuming activity.*
Waiting 30 minutes may be recommended only if the nitroglycerin is effective in relieving the chest pain.

D. *Keep extra nitroglycerin in an airtight and light-resistant bottle.*
This is excellent medication teaching, but it does not have the same urgency as seeking emergency care.

21. The nurse is providing discharge teaching for a client who is prescribed diltiazem (Cardizem). Which dietary instruction has the highest priority?

Rationales:

A. *Maintain a low-sodium diet.*
The client may need to restrict sodium intake, but it is not specific for Cardizem.

B. *Eat a banana each morning.*
If the client has low potassium, this should be recommended.

C. *Ingest high-fiber foods daily.*
This is an excellent teaching point to prevent constipation but it is not the highest priority.

D. *Avoid grapefruit products.*
Grapefruit should be avoided when taking calcium channel blockers because it can cause an increase in the serum drug level, predisposing the client to hypotension.

22. The nurse is teaching a young adult female who has a history of Raynaud's disease how to control her pain. What information should the nurse offer?

Rationales:

A. *Take oral analgesic at regularly spaced intervals.*
Pain is not always associated with Raynaud's disease, but rather the feeling of cold hands and fingers and pallor. If pain is sporadic or situational, it should not necessitate regular use of analgesia.

B. *Avoid extremes of heat and cold.*
In Raynaud's disease, vascular spasms of the hands/fingers are triggered by exposure to extremes of heat or cold, which causes the characteristic pallor and cold-to-touch symptoms of the upper extremities.

C. *Limit foods and fluids with caffeine.*
Caffeine is not the primary trigger of the episodes, but if the client notes that caffeine contributes to the blanching and coldness, caffeine should be avoided.

D. *Keep involved extremities in dependent position.*
This is not effective for the client with Raynaud's disease.

23. The nurse is planning care for a client who is admitted with thrombocytopenia. Which nursing diagnosis best addresses this client's problem?

Rationales:

A. *Infection, risk for*
This is indicated for a client with neutropenia.

B. *Injury, risk for bleeding*
Thrombocytopenia refers to a low platelet count. Platelets are essential for initiating the normal clotting mechanism. This client is at risk for injury and bleeding.

C. *Impaired nutrition, less than requirements*
Nutrition should be addressed to ensure adequate iron intake, but this is not the present problem.

D. *Fatigue*
Fatigue is a problem associated with anemia.

Medical/Surgical Respiratory

24. A client who is admitted with cancer of the larynx is scheduled for a laryngectomy tomorrow. What is the top learning need for the client tonight?

Rationales:

A. *Body image counseling*
This is a concern after surgery when the immediate life-threatening insult of cancer is assimilated and basic needs are met.

B. *Pain management expectations*
Pain relief expectations are a priority, but the inability to convey (communicate) a subjective symptom, such as pain, is the fear the client perceives first.

C. *Communication techniques*
A client who is in crisis and anticipating the immediate postoperative period is concerned with immediate needs, such as the ability to express, convey, and obtain intervention.

D. *Postoperative nutritional needs*
Nutrition is important to promote healing, but the ability to communicate one's subjective needs is a higher priority.

Psychiatric Nursing

25. A victim of a motor vehicle collision arrives in the emergency department dead on arrival. What action should the nurse implement to assist the spouse with this crisis?

Rationales:

A. *Ask if there are family, friends, or clergy to call.*
The nurse should help the spouse identify support systems and resources that are helpful while coping with a crisis situation, such as the sudden death of a spouse.

B. Talk about the former relationship with the spouse.
The spouse may be unable to process information during the crisis, and the nurse should focus on immediate needs for coping and support.

C. Provide education about the stages of grief and loss.
Educating the client about grief and loss is not an immediate priority in the crisis and should be provided after the spouse begins to cope with the crisis.

D. Assess the spouse's levels of anxiety.
Although the nurse should assess the spouse for anxiety, the immediate approach should include a directive approach to assist the spouse in dealing with the stressful event.

26. **The nurse is planning to lead a seminar for clinic and community health nurses on violence against women during pregnancy. Which statement describes an appropriate technique to assess for violence?**

Rationales:

A. Women should be assessed only if they are part of high-risk groups.
Violence against women occurs in all ethnic groups and at all income levels.

B. Women may be assessed in the presence of young children, but not intimate partners.
It is important to assess women without their partners present; it is also important that verbal children not be present, as they may repeat what is heard. Infants may be present.

C. Women should be assessed once during pregnancy.
Many women do not reveal violence the first time they are asked. As trust develops between nurse and client, the client may be more comfortable sharing her story. Also, violence may start later in the pregnancy.

D. <u>Women should be reassessed face to face by a nurse as the pregnancy progresses.</u>
More than one face-to-face interview elicits the highest reports of violence during pregnancy.

27. **The charge nurse reminds several clients on the mental health unit that breakfast is at 8 AM, medications are given at 9 AM, and group therapy sessions begin at 10 AM. Which treatment modality has been implemented?**

Rationales:

A. <u>Milieu therapy</u>
Milieu therapy uses resources and activities in the environment to assist with improving social functioning and activities of daily living.

B. Behavior modification
Behavior modification involves changing behaviors with positive and negative reinforcements to allow desired activities or remove privileges.

C. Peer therapy
Peer therapy is not a single therapeutic modality, but uses peers who are responsible for supporting, sharing, and compromising within their peer group and milieu.

D. Problem solving
Problem solving is used in crisis intervention and focuses on the problem identification and ways to return to prior levels of functioning.

28. **The nurse is accompanying a male client to x-ray when he becomes panic stricken at the elevator and states, "I can't get on that elevator." Which action should the nurse implement first?**

Rationales:

A. Ask one more staff member to ride the elevator.
One more staff member will not be able to mobilize the client to ride the elevator because he must first recognize his feelings about the phobia and accept the need to change his behavior.

B. Offer the antianxiety medication.
Offering an antianxiety medication may be needed to proceed with desensitization.

C. Begin desensitization about riding the elevator.
Desensitizing the client may be implemented, but first the client should identify his fears and recognize his anxiety.

D. <u>Affirm his fear about riding the elevator.</u>
The nurse should first validate and allow the client to affirm his anxiety and fears about riding the elevator. Then options to initiate desensitization may be considered.

29. **A male client who experiences frequent nightmares and somnambulism is found one night trying to strangle his roommate. Which action that the nurse should implement has the highest priority?**

Rationales:

A. Give the client a sedative or hypnotic.
Sleepwalking is more likely to occur when the client is fatigued, is anxious, and has received a hypnotic or sedative, but safety is the priority.

B. Administer an antipsychotic medication.
An antipsychotic medication is indicated if the client is psychotic and agitated, but the nurse should ensure the safety of both clients first.

C. <u>Move the client to a different room.</u>
The nurse should implement safety precautions immediately and move the client to a private room to protect both clients from harm or retaliation.

D. Process with both clients about the event.
Although both clients should talk about the incident, this is not an opportune time, and the clients should be separated to provide a safe environment.

30. **The nurse is updating the plan of care for a client who has a borderline personality disorder. Which intervention should be included with the nursing diagnosis of ineffective coping related to manipulation?**

Rationales:

A. <u>Refer the client's requests to one nurse.</u>
The best intervention is to provide consistency and avoid splitting by assigning the client to only one nurse.

B. *Avoid challenging inappropriate behavior.*
The nurse should assist the client to recognize manipulative behavior and set limits on manipulative behaviors as necessary.

C. *Limit client's contacts with other clients.*
Socialization should be encouraged to improve skills with others.

D. *Remove consequences for acting-out behavior.*
Firm limits with clear expectations and consequences are needed for clients with manipulation.

31. **A female adolescent is admitted to the mental health unit for anorexia nervosa. What is the nurse's priority intervention?**

Rationales:

A. *Teach about the importance of self-expression.*
Self-expression of feelings is important, but reestablishing normal eating habits and physiological integrity is the priority intervention.

B. *Supervise activities during the day.*
The nurse should monitor and supervise the client's activities to prevent bingeing, purging, or avoiding meals.

C. *Include in daily group therapy.*
The client should be included in daily groups, but the priority is physiological needs and monitoring meals.

D. *Facilitate social interactions with others.*
The client should be given opportunities to socialize, but monitoring activities during the day and especially meals is the priority.

32. **The charge nurse is planning the daily schedule for clients on the mental health unit. To which activity group should a male client who is manic be assigned?**

Rationales:

A. *Basketball game in the gym.*
The client should avoid any potential competitive physical activity, especially contact sports, that can stimulate aggressive acting-out.

B. *Jogging at least 1 mile.*
Jogging is the best activity for the client because it is a noncompetitive physical activity, which requires the use of large muscle groups that expend energy associated with mania.

C. *Ping-pong game with peer.*
The nurse should avoid assigning the client to any competitive activities that can frustrate the client and stimulate mood swings.

D. *Group therapy with the art therapist.*
A manic client may become disruptive and distracted in an art group, and physical energy using large muscle groups is more effective in expending energy.